SCRUFFY'S
PAWSITIVE
MISSION

SCRUFFY'S
PAWSITIVE
MISSION
ATTACKING PANIC DISORDER

by Scruffy and Patty Pleban

Temple Publishing LLC

Cleveland, OH

First Edition, First Printing, January, 2000
Temple Publishing, Cleveland, OH, www.templepublishing.com

The instructions and advice in this book are in no way intended
as a substitute for medical counseling. We advise the reader to consult
with his/her doctor or professional counselor before beginning
any type of self-help program. The author and the publisher
disclaim any liability or loss, personal or otherwise,
resulting from the information
or procedures in this book.

Printed in the United States of America

10 9 8 7 6 5 4 3 2 1

ISBN No. 1-58446-003-2

Illustrations
by Tudi Pleban

Book Layout & Cover Design
by Doreen M. Buck

DEDICATION

*"TO FLORENCE AND LEONARD PLEBAN
FOR THEIR INTUITION THAT I WOULD
HELP PATTY"*

—Scruffy

*"TO SCRUFFY AND MY PARENTS FOR
BRINGING HER INTO MY LIFE"*

—Patty

ACKNOWLEDGMENTS

God has given me many blessings in life and I thank Him. I think because of His infinite wisdom He knew I would need a lot of help with my life's journey and provided me with my family, friends, professionals and yes, even Scruffy.

My parents have given me their priceless gifts of faith, unconditional love, support, positive thinking, and humor. Most of all, they have instilled the importance of family. Tudi, Linny and Gary, your understanding, giving and caring natures helped me so very much, proving the strength of family is immeasurable.

I also want to thank my extended family. Your telephone calls, cards, prayers and words of encouragement were very important and meant so much. I wish to give a special thanks to Aunt Clara and Candy for their endless support.

My significant other, Vernon Wherry, whose love, devotion, understanding, strength and confidence have all been invaluable. You have taught me so many of life's lessons. You are my hero.

My love and gratefulness to forever friends Livie, Dan, Brenna, Joann, Edie, Charlene, Terry, Margie, John, Karen, Debbie, Marion and Mrs. Ferguson who were always there. To my new friends Bill, Carol, Dorothy, Laura, Dawn, Jan, Mary Ann, Vicki, Delsie, Mark and my Buhl Club family who have all touched my life and given me the wealth of their friendships.

My heartfelt thanks to Drs. Demetrious Lagoutaris, Mary De Angelis and Joseph Conti, who have been blessed with the special gifts of healing. Our world is a better place because of their compassion.

I am so grateful for all of the prayers from the religious order of nuns in Erie, Pennsylvania, Father Justin Ratajszak, Father Ted Carter, and the late Father Joseph Marinack and Father James Eliot.

To those who passed before this book was published, Anna Mae Lynn, Florine Reda, Dolly Hughes, Mary and Nick Roscoe, Leo Buscalia and John Fridley, thank you for your inspiration of life.

My sincere appreciation to Maggi, who was there from the start to finish of this book. Your countless hours of help, support and friendship are all true signs of a cherished friend.

My admiration to Dr. Daniel Baker, Baker Animal Hospital, Dr. James Prueter of the Veterinary Referral Clinic, the Humane Society and Pet Therapy Groups who realize that pets have a very positive affect on our lives.

I am very fortunate to have Betty Wasiloff in my life. She believed in me and was determined to see *Scruffy's Pawsitive Mission* help others.

PREFACE

When I had my first full-blown panic attack, I felt the experience was unique only to me. Not only did I feel out of control, but I was almost positive I had lost my mind. I felt ashamed, embarrassed and that I had let down so many people in my life. Little did I know at the time that it is estimated that between three to six million adults, in America alone, suffer from panic disorders that severely restrict and impair work, family and social relationships.

After many years of isolating myself, and with the help of therapy, I decided that before I rejoined the outside world I would be open about what I had experienced. The results led to this book. It seemed people I came in contact with either wanted me to write or talk to someone they knew was agoraphobic. Many of the people themselves had experienced panic. I decided to write about my experience, but I wanted it to be non-threatening and desensitized, even though I know it is a serious illness. This book should not replace professional help.

Scruffy, who came to live with me at the worst time of my life, became the author of this book. My story is told through her eyes to lighten up a heavy topic. She relates how, when one member of a family has panic disorder, the entire family is affected by the condition. Many studies are being done to show the effects pets have with the health of humans. Results have already proven pets can decrease blood pressure, lead the blind, alert humans of an oncoming seizure, and improve mental well being in nursing homes.

I feel in my heart Scruffy was sent to me. Her unconditional love, help and support were immeasurable. I wanted to share Scruffy with you in the hope that her "pawsitive mission" will also help you or someone you love.

CHAPTER ONE

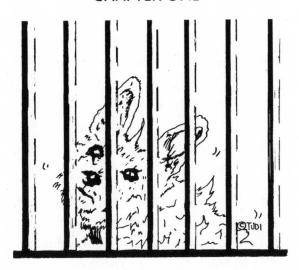

Human beings do not realize the responsibility and commitment that goes "paw in paw" with being a dog. I think that is why we were given four paws to handle it all. Then I am convinced Our Creator looked at us and knew of the unconditional love we would give and gave us the name of DOG. That in itself is the ultimate responsibility since it is His name spelled backwards.

It was late fall in 1984 and I was ready for a new assignment. What it would be I was not told. Just that — I would know. What a day to move on. Humans would say it was raining cats and dogs. All I knew was the rain was pouring down and running into my big brown eyes. My blonde hair, even in the best conditions, is unruly and wiry. Now it was getting dirty because my short legs were stepping through some very deep puddles. I don't know why humans would build sidewalks so close to my body. I usually have a curl on top of my head. I just know it was plastered to my scalp. Humans talk about bad hair days. Why couldn't I have been bigger like a German Shepherd or a Great Dane instead of my mere fifteen pounds? I was also starting not to smell so good — even to myself. Gosh, I am getting really cold. Why did I pick today to move on?

I have heard from other dogs what can happen when you're out on your own. Dogcatchers and human beings that do not look where they are driving are the biggest threats. Then of course I have to watch out for mean humans and dogs. I am really getting hungry, tired, and cold. There has been a van that seems to be checking me out. It is STOPPING. Well, what the heck, the female human looks kind and I am exhausted. Who knows, maybe through this human I'll meet who I am supposed to help, and riding in this van sure beats walking.

I am really one lucky dog. This female human is so very nice. She introduced herself as Gerda and said she would call me Scruffy since I didn't have any identification. I know I don't look my best but had she been through my experiences before she rescued me, would she look any better? I know I made the right choice in not running away from her. I wonder where she is taking me?

We stopped at a house that had a high fence surrounding the back yard. Gerda carried me into the house and there were all these other dogs to greet me. Before I got to mingle, Gerda cleaned me up and gave me a shot. I do trust her; she seems to know what she is doing and it didn't even hurt. Well, maybe just a little. Now I get to eat and have a nice cold drink. I think I will wait until tomorrow to talk to the other dogs. I am so tired. I just want to sleep for a while.

I felt so much better when I got up. I found out from the other dogs that we had one thing in common. We were all in transit. Like myself, there were a couple of dogs that were looking for humans to help. Some of the others were looking for new homes because their humans had to move. What really tugged at my heart though, were the dogs that were there because they had been abused. So, I listened to their stories. I just shook my head and wondered what this world was coming to. How can most humans be so nice while others are so cruel? What happens to humans to make them like that? I KNOW they are not born cruel.

Gerda, the others told me, was one of the most compassionate humans they had ever met. She was head of the Humane Society, which helped us animals with our rights. She was not like some of the other humans who ran other agencies. There, if you did not find a home in three days, you were one dead dog. Instead, she matched dogs and humans very carefully and took all the time needed to accomplish this task. What a very special human she is. I even found out her phone number had the name NOAH in it. We all know the big job he had with the animals.

Gerda took me to the Baker Animal Hospital. I was not sick but even animals need preventive care. There I met Terry, Dawn, Mindy, Robin, Jill, Michelle and Sharon who all helped Dr. Baker in one way or another. They played with me and talked to me while I was waiting my turn. They also were very impressed with the curl on top of my head.

The minute I saw Dr. Baker I knew I could trust him not to hurt me. I liked him. Anyone who goes to school for so many years to learn so much about animals has to have a kind heart. I am going to be spayed, which is the first step for adoption. I never knew how many unwanted animals there were. Dr. Baker looks at me like I am special. He tells me how smart I am. I think he knows I am looking for someone to help. There is a dialogue between us like others who don't speak a common language — through eye contact. Yes, I like Dr. Baker. He is my friend. I hope when I find my new home he can be my doctor so I can see him.

This adoption process takes a long time. I never knew how many other dogs were looking for new homes. Gerda has been so nice to me, but I know someone is waiting for my help and I must find this human. I decided to jump the fence in the backyard to resume my search. This adventure was cut short when the police picked me up. I really liked hanging out at the Police Station. They were all very nice to me. They tried to find a home for me among themselves. Some had dogs already and the others lived in homes where dogs were not permitted. Maybe they would let me become a Police Dog. I like riding in cars. I like helping humans. It is really confusing sometimes when you don't know what you should do with your life. So I asked for guidance from the Creator. The next thing I knew I was back with Gerda.

The news came shortly after that a human was coming to see me. The lady was very nice and took me home to her son. He was autistic. I could help here, but I did not feel I could help him enough. This was not who I was supposed to be helping.

Although we dogs do verbalize our feelings, humans do not always understand because we speak a different language. I have heard humans who speak the same language sometimes have trouble communicating with each other. I had to let these humans know I was not supposed to be here. My dilemma caused me to throw up. After a couple of days of this, the female human knew she had her hands full with her autistic son and did not need a dog with a weak stomach. Back to Gerda I went.

Gerda was all excited to see me. I thought by now she might think I was a troublemaker, but she just knew that I was not where I was supposed to be. She looked at me and smiled saying "Scruffy, another family has called about you. They were very impressed that you were housebroken and happy you were small. They had read your ad in the newspaper and I told them you were already adopted. I knew I had other doggies that needed homes so I told them to come over. I did not know you would be back. I felt you, Scruffy, had a special mission to do. I also know you will know what it is soon. You're very unique, Scruffy." Gerda went on to tell me Dr. Pleban was looking for a dog for his daughter, who was suffering from agoraphobia, a debilitating form of panic disorder.

The daughter lived by herself and everyone was very concerned about her because she would not leave her house. This had been going on for years. Can you believe that? Staying in your house and not going anywhere — for years. Well, I guess everyone was concerned about her because she used to be a very active person.

Her landlady said her family could get her a dog, even though she had a strict rule about no pets. This is it! I just know it! So I will not be going for rides in the car. Sometimes you have to make sacrifices. This is whom I am supposed to help. I do not know that much about panic disorder or agoraphobia, but I will learn.

Just then the doorbell rang. That always caused much excitement amongst us dogs. We all would bark and jump up and down knowing this could be our new family coming for us. I see a male human talking to Gerda and with him is a female human. The male is of average height, but you can tell that is the only average thing about him. He has on a heavy black coat and hat which he removes uncovering his silver-gray hair. His face is very kind and his eyes sparkle with confidence. I could tell he was a thoughtful human and not just because he was here looking for a dog for his daughter. The female human with him is his youngest daughter. She came along because she is a real dog lover and wants to find the right one for her sister. She is petite with blonde hair like me. I know I would fit in this family. Her face was radiant and she was cute, too. I will never forget the first time I heard her infectious laugh. I heard Gerda say, "Well, come on in and take a look at the dogs, Dr. Pleban and Tudi.

What does she mean the dogs? I know they called about me. This is it. I know I can help out here. How do I get them to pick me over the other dogs? Here they come. They are sitting down looking at all of us dogs. I could not stand it anymore. I knew this was my mission—my new assignment. I jumped up on Dr. Pleban's lap and gave him a big kiss. His eyes caught mine and I heard the words I had been waiting to hear. "This is the dog."

Gerda said my name was Scruffy and she thought I was the right choice. So I left Gerda and the other dogs and went with Dr. Pleban and Tudi, never looking back. I had to look ahead.

I had a big challenge waiting for me but I was ready!

Once in the car Tudi did her imitation of a barking dog for me. I gave her a big kiss because I knew she was trying to make me feel welcomed. Yes, I made the right choice. I am ready to get started on my mission.

CHAPTER TWO

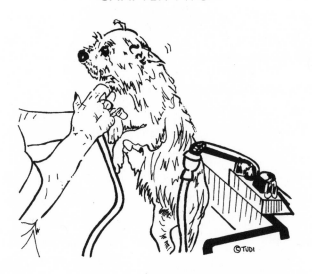

Well, I thought I was as ready as I could be, but Flo did not think I was ready enough. Flo is Dr. Pleban's wife. Now this female human is a real dog lover. She drew me a bath in the stationary tub to scrub me up, and never stopped talking the whole time. She relayed to me, that it was Christmas Eve Day and I was going to be a present for Patty. Patty had gone to school for merchandising and had been in the buying program for a major department store when she claimed she started feeling strange sensations. That was four years ago. These feelings are so overwhelming that she will not leave her house. Patty has been experiencing these feelings a lot longer. At first there was so much time between episodes she thought each time would be the last. Therefore, until four years ago she continued to go through the motions of living her life as if she were in control. No one who knew her would have ever thought she had a problem.

Patty was flying back home from a trip she had taken when she could not hide these feelings. The air travel time was not long. She had flown this trip many times before so it was not a new location or a new experience. She had always loved flying, especially taking off. Sure, with all the flying she had done there had been some stormy weather and she would become anxious, but not like this. It was not even storming. It was a smooth flight. She also knew that each time she had flown lately it was becoming increasingly harder to get on the plane. She really had to force herself to fly. On this particular flight, her feelings had gone beyond anxious. She was experiencing sheer panic. Butterflies in her stomach, being warm all over and muscle tension were all familiar sensations. These were accompanied, however, with the need to escape, tightness in her chest, the feeling of doom, dizziness, nausea, and concern for losing control. She felt very detached and frantic with these weird sensations and feelings.

Every sound and movement of the plane was magnified to its fullest extent in her mind. She started thinking WHAT-IF the nuts and bolts on this plane are loose? The plane is going to crash! The pilots' lives are at stake. They would not want to crash but WHAT-IF they had bad home lives and had nothing to live for? The wings look like they are shaking! WHAT-IF they fall off? The engines are making noises! WHAT-IF they catch on fire? Patty asked the flight attendant what was happening. She said, "The flight was on time and was going smooth." Patty asked to see another flight attendant, and another until all had confirmed what the first attendant had said. She then asked to have them land the plane so she could get off. Then she said she wanted her parachute. The flight attendant told her there wasn't a parachute, but a flotation device. Through clinched teeth Patty said, "What do you mean no parachute? What good is a flotation device, we are not even flying over water!" She demanded to see the pilot. She pleaded and begged him to land the plane now. He told her the plane would be landing in a matter of minutes at its destination.

There is a response called "fight or flight," but I think Patty took this literally. If you have a lot of stress and do not know how to cope with it, your body becomes aroused because it is being bombarded with anxiety-producing stimuli. Nature's purpose in allowing the body to become aroused is protection. When faced with sudden danger, you become physically ready to react by either fighting the stressor or fleeing from it. When the brain puts into action what is called the "fight or flight" response, it releases hormones known as corticosteroids. These powerful hormones constrict the blood vessels in the peripheral parts of the body in order to drive blood into the brain and deep down into the large muscles for added strength. The heart pounds, digestion shuts down, breathing increases and muscles tighten.

The "fight or flight" response progresses in three stages. The first stage is the ALARM STAGE as I already described. If the emergency is suddenly resolved, and you escape from the danger, your body reverses the alarm stage and sends the physical conditions back to normal. If the threat persists, however, a second stage, known as the RESISTANCE STAGE, appears. The physiological responses such as muscle tension and digestive conditions become fixed. If the body is forced to maintain a stage of resistance for too long a period or if the threat is repeated often enough, a final EXHAUSTION STAGE develops. The body can no longer adapt to the threat, and the systems collapse. [1]

"Patty never flew again after this incident." In my mind, as Flo is telling me this, I'm thinking that the whole airline industry is grateful for that. So I learned flying was the first thing Patty let go of in her life. This was the start of her avoidance.

Malls and large shopping centers were next. This was a gradual process three years after the flying incident. Patty eventually would only go into stores at the mall that had a direct outside exit. Since she was in merchandising, the thought of going to work and having to stay there in a large store became so overwhelming she left her job.

Grocery stores and churches were finally the last two places she avoided. Both were gradual, going to a smaller store each time the feeling of panic took over. Finally, Patty was doing her shopping in a neighborhood store with three aisles. Flo said Patty had even tried taking people shopping with her. That way if she had to leave someone could check out for her. She had also gone to four different churches until even the smallest chapel became too overwhelming.

I could understand how Patty thought if going into places causes these feelings—why not try drive-thrus. So everything she could find—drug stores, banks, and even some mini-mart stores—she drove through. Eventually these feelings of panic started taking over when she was in line at the drive-thrus. She especially felt panicky when she was pinned in and could not go forward or back up. Many times, she would circle a drive-thru until there wasn't a line. These feelings were now starting to be associated with the car and driving. She did not know what was happening to her. Was she losing her mind? Going crazy? The only place she felt safe anymore was at her home. That is where she has been for four years now.

Flo was done making me beautiful. I looked better than I ever had. I smelled good, too. All that scrubbing made me feel really good. Then I was blow-dried, which made my hair fluffier than ever. Flo really knows how to treat a dog. I wonder if she can give me my bath all the time. Leonard and Tudi came down to the den to check me out. This was good for my ego.

"How pretty you are," Tudi said.

Leonard said I was beautiful and reaffirmed I was the right choice.

CHAPTER THREE

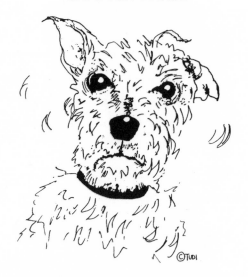

Flo, Leonard, and Tudi were busy the whole day. There sure is a lot to this Christmas Eve stuff at this house. They were doing things like last minute shopping. I did not want anyone to think I was eavesdropping, but I did hear that since Scruffy was now in the family she had to have some Christmas presents.

After humans buy these presents, they wrap them in pretty paper and tie ribbons on them. Then they are placed under a big tree that has lights and other shiny things on it. They look like balls. This tree is like trees I have seen outside, but never with all this stuff on it.

The smells in the house were making me hungry. There was food in both ovens and on top of the stove. There is going to be lots of food after church. The way I understand it, the order is church, presents, and food with family and friends stopping by to visit. Why can't food be first? The family goes to church together, that is everyone except Patty. They will pick her up afterwards. She has not been able to go with them for years and I know they miss her.

Someone is at the door. I thought company did not come until after church and presents, but when it was time for the food.

Maybe I got things mixed up and it is time to eat.

Leonard said, "Linny and Gary, meet Scruffy."

Linny is Patty's other sister and Gary is her husband. Linny was tall. In fact, she was the tallest human in this family. Her coloring was fair and her hair was dark. Her dark eyes had a look of inquisitiveness and hope as she looked at me.

Gary, on the other hand, had a devilish twinkle in his eyes, and that was the only thing that gave him away. He was distinguished looking with his mustache and full beard. When he spoke everything was very pronounced. So if you didn't see that twinkle in his eye you would think he was very reserved and formal.

As Flo and Leonard did some last minute Christmas things before they left for church, Linny and Tudi took me down to the den. Off the den was a laundry room where I would stay until everyone came home. The room was very nice with lots of throw rugs so I would be comfortable if I laid down. I had water, food, and some treats. I did not mind being confined, but I was housebroken. Maybe I had to prove myself. Oh well, after all we were just getting to know each other.

Linny said, "Tudi, I hope Scruffy is the answer."

Tudi replied, "I really think Scruffy is the answer. Look at that face. It's like she already understands that she has a mission to do."

Linny said, "You know, Tudi, Patty has not had a dog since we were young. Suppose she doesn't take to Scruffy?"

Tudi answered, "I'm not worried. Scruffy has an air of confidence about her. I have a feeling she will not give up. Look at her, she looks like she is saying 'I can handle this challenge'."

I listened as Linny and Tudi recalled the past five years. This was not eavesdropping—this was research. They recalled when Patty first went to the doctors to receive a complete check up. The sensations she felt while these unexplained feelings were happening were so physical.

Much later everyone would learn that, according to Dr. Arthur B. Hardy, "There are several common physiological reactions that one can experience during attacks of anxiety or panic. Although they produce uncomfortable feelings, all are NORMAL, NATURAL body reactions that are NOT DANGEROUS in any way."[1]

THE RESPIRATORY SYSTEM

"There is frequently a tightness in the chest, which gives the feeling of being short of breath. This condition leads to 'over-breathing' or hyperventilation, a very common symptom of anxiety. Hyperventilation is part of the normal fear reaction of preparing the body for flight. Its purpose is to oxygenate the blood, but sometimes, as a result of breathing excessively and rapidly, too much oxygen (O2) is taken in and, at the same time, too much carbon dioxide (CO2) is breathed out. The excess of C2 (carbon) combined with the relative shortage of CO2 can lead to feelings of light-headedness, dizziness, depersonalization, a tingling sensation in fingers and toes, a numbness around the mouth, and if hyperventilation continues, spasms of leg or arm muscles. One of the most preliminary and effective ways to prevent hyperventilation from occurring is to breathe with your mouth closed. Breathing through the nose reduces the intake of C2 considerably and also limits the amount of CO2 (carbon dioxide) exhaled.

THE CARDIOVASCULAR SYSTEM
(HEART AND BLOOD VESSELS)

"The cardiovascular system is highly responsive to emotion. The heart can slow down, speed up, beat heavily; blood pressure can increase or decrease; the blood vessels can constrict, impeding the flow of blood, or they can dilate and increase the flow of blood. Dilation of the small arteries produces a sensation of warmth to the skin, increases the flow of blood to the surface of the body, and causes a drop in blood pressure, which produces a feeling of light-headedness, dizziness, or instability. The sensation causes the person to worry that he might fall or faint or lose control of himself. The heart speeds up and beats heavily, reactions called tachycardia and heart palpitations. These conditions are not dangerous, but they are uncomfortable and can arouse the worry that something has gone wrong with one's heart. The same reaction can be created by injections of adrenaline. During attacks of anxiety, the nervous system causes extra adrenaline to be produced.

THE GASTROINTESTINAL SYSTEM
(STOMACH AND BOWEL)

"The gastrointestinal (GI) system, which includes the mouth and throat, is also very responsive to emotional stimuli. Two main reactions can occur: the GI tract can be stimulated to secrete fluid and become active, or it can stop secreting and stop its activity. Typically, the mouth becomes dry, which makes it hard to swallow, and there is a tightening of the muscles in the throat. This gives rise to the fear that the throat will constrict and cut off air and possibly prevents the eating of solid food.

THE SKIN

"Even the skin is emotionally reactive. With the warmth also comes perspiration. There is generalization sweating, but it is more pronounced on the palms of the hands and on the upper lip and brow of the face. The warmth and blushing are due to dilation of the small arteries under the skin close to the surface.

THE MUSCULAR SYSTEM

"The muscles respond by increased tension—shaky tremors in the mild form and jerky reactions in the stronger form. The muscles may become tight and tense; they may ache from fatigue, and become sore and painful. There are other reactions that can be measured; but we don't always recognize these as feelings, such as restlessness, urges to run or urges to hit or scream, in any event, the muscular system too is prepared for flight."[2]

Even though Patty had so many physical symptoms, her check up and tests revealed she had nothing physically wrong. It was then suggested that she consult a psychiatrist. Society still hadn't accepted therapy as they do now. The first time she went she was nervous. Therapy still had a stigma attached to it. Leonard went with her. While they were in the office waiting room, two children were playing games with their grandmother. Their mother was with the doctor. As Patty watched the children play, the one child said to the other, "Are you crazy, why did you do that?" Patty cringed, as the word CRAZY seemed to echo in her mind. Was she really crazy? How did this happen?

Her first visit with the psychiatrist was the start of a nightmare. She had nothing to compare with a visit to the psychiatrist. When Patty told the doctor of her symptoms he said, "You are having these feelings because you are involved with a married man."

She looked at him in disbelief and said she wasn't.

He told her he had seen this many times with women in merchandising.

Patty told him she was not even dating anyone. He replied that until she was honest with him, she would continue to have these feelings. He then prescribed medication.

Patty thought the medicine would take these feelings away.

Each visit to this psychiatrist went the same way. "Are you still having the same sensations?" He would ask.

"Yes," Patty replied.

"Then we will also add this medication," he would say.

This went on until Patty said to him, "I'm not used to taking so much medication. I am getting very confused. Please write down the names of the pills and when I should take them."

The end of her sessions with this psychiatrist came when Leonard had called Patty one Saturday morning. She did not know who he was. He went over to her house and she was totally confused. Leonard asked what she was taking. Patty showed him the long list of medications and the times they were to be taken as directed by the doctor. Leonard was appalled. How could anyone prescribe all this medication? He made his feelings known to the doctor.

The feelings were worse; Patty saw another psychiatrist. This one diagnosed her as a manic-depressive.

Since certain medications and combinations of medications can cause this effect, it was no wonder she was extremely depressed considering what she had just been through. This doctor gave her medication that blurred her vision so badly that she couldn't focus at all. Then prescribed a pill to counteract the pill that was impairing her vision. He also gave her medication for her "supposed" manic depression.

Patty was now in the depths of depression. How could all this be happening to her, she thought? She had seen two psychologists and both thought it best for her to be institutionalized.

Despair began to take over and Patty even tried to take her life three times. She was in complete disbelief when her family and friends became angry with her and told her how much she had to live for. In her mind, she thought everyone would be so much better off without her to have to worry about. She was hurting. She saw no light at the end of the tunnel. She didn't even know how this happened to her, let alone how to fix it. Patty felt that no parents, sisters or friends should have to go through what she was putting them through.

Meeting Dr. Lagoutaris was the only good thing that had happened to her for a long time. The old adage about the third time being a charm was true because this was now her third psychiatrist. He did not agree with the other psychologists who treated Patty and was opposed to her being institutionalized. The doctor went on to say Patty was suffering from agoraphobia, a panic disorder. Dr. Lagoutaris told Patty she would get better. He compared the process to climbing a mountain. There will be times you climb so high and there will be times you slide backwards. In your struggle to reach the top of your mountain, determination will help. All your efforts will be worth it because at the top of your mountain is your castle.

Linny and Tudi recalled they were relieved when, at last, Dr. Lagoutaris identified what was wrong with Patty. Knowing that there is a name for what you are experiencing, instead of thinking you are going crazy, had to be of some consolation to her. The whole family had questions and discovered their questions had answers.

WHAT IS PANIC DISORDER?

"Panic disorder is a serious health problem in this country. At least 1.6 percent of adult Americans, or three million people will have panic disorder at some time in their lives.

"The disorder is strikingly different from other types of anxiety in that panic attacks are so sudden, appear to be unprovoked, and are often disabling.

"Once someone has had a panic attack—for example, while driving, shopping in a crowded store, or riding in an elevator-he or she may develop irrational fears, called phobias, about these situations and begin to avoid them. Eventually, the pattern of avoidance and level of anxiety about another attack may reach the point where the individual with panic disorder may be unable to drive or even step out of the house. At this stage, the person is said to have panic disorder with agoraphobia. Thus, panic disorder can have as serious an impact on a person's daily life as other major illnesses—unless the individual receives effective treatment.

WHAT ARE THE SYMPTOMS
OF A PANIC ATTACK?

"The symptoms of a panic attack appear suddenly, without any apparent cause. They may include:

● Racing or pounding heartbeat

● Chest pains

● Dizziness, light-headedness, nausea

● Difficulty in breathing

● Tingling or numbness in the hands

● Flushes or chills

● Dreamlike sensations or perceptual distortions

● Terror—a sense that something unimaginably horrible is about to occur and one is powerless to prevent it

● Fear of losing control and doing something embarrassing

● Fear of dying [3]

Another periodical lists some of the same symptoms and others:

● Shortness of breath or smothering sensations

● Dizziness, unsteady feelings or faintness

● Palpitations or accelerated heart rate

- Trembling or shaking

- Sweating

- Choking

- Nausea or abdominal distress

- Depersonalization or derealization

- Numbness or tingling sensations

- Flushes (hot flashes) or chills

- Chest pains or discomfort

- Fear of dying

- Fear of going crazy or doing something uncontrolled [4]

"A panic attack typically lasts for several minutes and is one of the most distressing conditions that a person can experience. Most who have one attack will have others. When someone has repeated attacks, or feels severe anxiety about having another attack, he or she is (said) to have a panic disorder." [5]

"Agoraphobia not only includes the panic disorder symptoms but goes one step further in that an agoraphobic experiences the fear of being in places or situations from which escape might be difficult (or embarrassing) or in which help might not be available in the event of a panic attack." [6]

IS PANIC DISORDER SERIOUS?

"Yes, panic disorder is real and potentially disabling, but it can be controlled with specific treatments. Because of the disturbing symptoms that accompany panic disorder, it may be mistaken for heart disease or some other life-threatening medical illness. People frequently go to hospital emergency rooms when they are having panic attacks, and extensive medical tests may be performed to rule out these other conditions.

"Medical personnel generally attempt to reassure the panic attack patient that he or she is not in great danger. But these efforts at reassurance can sometimes add to the patient's difficulties. If the doctors use expressions such as 'nothing serious,' 'all in your head,' or 'nothing to worry about,' this may give the incorrect impression that there is no real problem and that treatment is not possible or necessary.

WHAT IS THE TREATMENT
FOR PANIC DISORDER?

"Thanks to research, there are a variety of treatments available, including several effective medications, and also specific forms of psychotherapy. Often, a combination of psychotherapy and medications produces good results.

"In addition, people with panic disorder may need treatment for other emotional problems. Depression has often been associated with panic disorder, as have alcohol and drug abuse.

Recent research also suggests that suicide attempts are more frequent in people with panic disorder. Fortunately, these problems associated with panic disorder can be overcome effectively, just like panic disorder itself.

"Tragically, many people with panic disorder do not seek or receive treatment. To encourage recognition and treatment of panic disorder, the National Institute of Mental Health is sponsoring a major information campaign to acquaint the public and health care professionals with this disorder. National Institute of Mental Health is the agency of the U.S. Government responsible for improving the mental health of the American people by supporting research on the brain and mental disorders and by increasing public understanding of these conditions and their treatment.

WHAT HAPPENS IF PANIC DISORDER IS NOT TREATED?

"Panic disorder tends to continue for months or years. While it typically begins in young adulthood, in some people the symptoms may arise earlier or later in life. If left untreated, it may worsen to the point where the person's life is seriously affected by panic attacks and by attempts to avoid or conceal them. In fact, many people have had problems with friends and family or lost jobs while struggling to cope with panic disorder. There may be periods of spontaneous improvement in the disorder, but it does not usually go away unless the person receives treatments designed specifically to help people with panic disorder.

WHAT CAUSES PANIC DISORDER?

"According to one theory of panic disorder, the body's normal 'alarm system'—the set of mental and physical mechanisms that allow a person to respond to threat—tends to be triggered unnecessarily when there is no danger. Scientists don't know exactly why this happens, or why some people are more susceptible to the problem than others. Panic disorder has been found to run in families, and this may mean that inheritance (genes) plays a strong role in determining who will get it. However, many people who have no family history of the disorder develop it. Often the first attacks are triggered by physical illnesses, a major life stressor, or perhaps medications that increase activity in the part of the brain involved in fear reactions."[7]

"So, we do know more than when this all started with Patty," Linny said.

"The key is getting Patty to want to help herself," replied Tudi.

"Mom and Dad are calling us. It must be time to go to church." Linny said, "Let's go pray Scruffy will help Patty."

"God knows we have tried everything else," Tudi said as

she gave me a kiss on top of my head, said she was counting on me and closed the laundry room door.

I sure did get a BIG assignment. This will be as important as the job police dogs and seeing eye dogs have. If love alone could make Patty better, she surely would have been better by now with these humans. Maybe the humans should have taken me to church so I could do a little praying myself. I don't know how, but I will help her.

CHAPTER FOUR

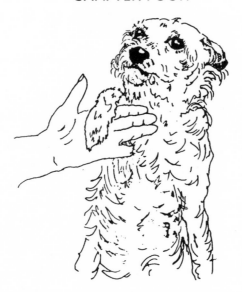

I hear voices upstairs. I wonder if they are home. What if it is a burglar and he eats all the food that Flo prepared? I started barking. I figured I could not go wrong. If it were a burglar I would scare him off. If it were my new family they would be impressed that I am such a good guard dog. That will be good for some points. I hope that while I was resting I didn't mess up my hair too much. I wonder if the big red bow Flo put on me after my bath is straight. Someone is coming downstairs. I will sit pretty and tilt my head to one side. Humans always think that is "so cute."

"So you are Scruffy. I have heard so much about you. I am Patty."

What she didn't know was I had heard about her too.

"I guess we are going to be roommates," she said with tears in her eyes.

Humans are sure different than dogs. We cry when we are in pain. They cry when they are hurt, sad, in pain, and happy. I think Patty was crying because she was all of these. I gave her lots of kisses as she opened the door and bent down to hug me. Patty, like the others, was not very tall. She was, however, very round, which made her look like a ball. Her hair was the same color as mine. Her eyes were very blue and showed me that she possessed love, tenderness, warmth, but also felt uneasiness, apprehension and concern. No, she could not hide her feelings with those eyes.

Everyone came downstairs to join in our meeting. Leonard and Tudi told Patty how they knew I was the right dog. Flo said how good I was during my bath and how smart I was because I seemed to understand everything she told me. What did she mean, "seemed"? I understood. Linny and Gary looked on hoping Patty would give me a chance. Little did they know I was determined to make this work.

Christmas Eve at this house is very special. There is so much laughing, caring, and love. There were lots of presents too. I got so many presents myself and I had only been here less than twenty-four hours. There were all different kinds of good dog treats, a new dog collar, toys, dog dishes, and even a sweater. I think I hit the jackpot with these humans. I can't let the moment make me forget why I was sent here. I do have a job to do. I stayed as close to Patty as I could. If she was sitting, I was beside her. If she got up to go to another part of the house, I followed her. And I don't think I have to tell you I was right there when she ate. Flo sure is a good cook. Then, that night when she slept I nestled right up to her to let her know I was there—I cared and would help in any way I could. I loved her already and knew soon that she would love me too.

As I cuddled there beside her, exhausted after such a big day, my mind was racing. I thought again about the love in this family. I also thought about how they had all in so many ways, tried to help Patty get better. It was at that time the thought came into my head. I can only help Patty to want to help her-self. She will be the one who has to do it. I will be there for her, but it is up to her.

Patty and I went home to her safe place the next day. The two-story brown house had white shutters on the windows. Since the house was built in the late 1870's, two additions had been built off the original house. They served as two apart-ments, one for Mrs. Ferguson, the landlady, the other for an-other family. I could see where Patty would feel safe here. Once inside, the first thing I saw was a fireplace. It didn't look like it had been used lately. Then I remembered Patty would not have been able to go out to get the wood. No, once inside, that is where she stayed. The windows had sheers and drapes cover-

ing them and over the covered door and windows Patty also
placed afghans to shut out the outside world. I would have to
do something about this because I love looking outside.

Christmas is just not celebrated in one day. The celebration
goes on for over a week with friends who visit. I liked it a lot
because everyone who came to visit brought me presents. When
humans come to visit, you have extra food to share with them.
I learned quickly that if I stared at them, they usually gave me
something. I also learned that it was not right to keep jumping
up or barking while they ate. Humans do not like that. No, I
just keep my big brown eyes fixed on them and throw in an
occasional wink which really gets to them.

Livie, Dan, and Brenna had come to visit. Livie had been
Patty's best friend for years. Dan was her husband and Brenna,
their daughter, was Patty's godchild. I could tell that Livie and
Patty shared a very special and loving friendship. Panic disorder and the agoraphobia had touched Patty's whole family; they
became very guarded in what they said to her. Livie, on the
other paw, was as close as any sister could be, and she also dared
to take more chances in what she said to Patty. She was very
encouraging but also very emphatic that Patty had to fight this.
Livie told her there were humans who were dying from diseases who would welcome the fight that Patty had to have to
get better. "You can do it," she kept saying.

When the two of them went into the kitchen, I heard Patty
telling Livie the panic attacks were even happening now here at

home in her safe place. She also told Livie that right before Christmas she began experiencing panic attacks when she was talking on the telephone and that she would have to hang up. I had not been around that long, but I already knew Patty liked talking on the telephone. After all, it was her only link to the outside world.

Just as she had felt safe in her safe place, home, Patty had safe humans she felt comfortable with. There, of course, were her family and Livie. Also, I had heard her talking a lot to Terry, a friend she had met in college. They talked about the "good old days" when they did not seem to have a care in the world. Terry knew that Patty's condition had worsened because before Patty would go visit Terry and her family if they came to get her. She wouldn't visit anymore. I could tell that Terry was very supportive. There was also Edie. She had gone to high school with Patty and was her roommate in college. When they were on the telephone one time I heard Patty say to Edie that her whole world had been so different before. She went on to tell Edie when she was in merchandising she always had a suitcase ready to go anywhere. She woke up in the mornings already knowing what and where she would be going even after working twelve-hour days. She continued saying her list of friends had dwindled and that was understandable considering how many excuses she made for not attending weddings, christenings, birthday parties, and funerals. This was because she was embarrassed to tell everyone the real truth. Patty also said she felt some of her friends who did know couldn't deal with it and may have been concerned they could get something like this. After all, everyone has something that makes him or her feel uncomfortable at times and some avoided her. Now she said, "I don't even like myself because of this. I, who was in such good physical shape, at least when this started, am now wearing size eighteen maternity clothes. I used to be a size seven/eight. How could this be happening to me, Edie?" I heard Patty ask, as tears rolled down her face.

Then I heard some hope in Patty's voice as she said, "I never thought of it like that, Edie," and she thanked her and hung up the telephone.

"Scruffy, do you know what Edie just said?" Patty asked me. She said, "Just like when I was in shape and going everywhere, I never thought anything like this would ever happen to me. There will be a time when you look back at what is happening to you now and you will know it happened, but you won't believe it. Oh, Scruffy, that would be so wonderful if Edie was right, wouldn't it?"

A few days after Christmas came New Year's Eve. Patty told me Mrs. Ferguson was celebrating this holiday with us. I was told this is where 1984 would end and a brand new year, 1985, would start. Mrs. Ferguson was a very good friend to Patty and she was also the landlady. She had given Flo and Leonard special permission for me to come and help Patty because she didn't allow pets in her rentals. Mrs. Ferguson always spent Christmas out of town with her family, but the past few years had made it a point to return so she and Patty could celebrate the New Year together. This Mrs. Ferguson sounded very special. She would even be bringing hats and noisemakers to make the night a little more festive. Patty told me how she had been so very kind by always encouraging her to fight the affliction. She assured her that she could call day or night. Mrs. Ferguson was the person Patty had taken with her when she went shopping in case she had to leave the store suddenly. She was also the one who would go into the store while Patty waited in the car when she was still driving.

When Mrs. Ferguson came I gave her lots of kisses. I made sure she knew I was very glad to meet her. After all, she had bent the rules for me. Patty was right. This white-haired female human, with the milky smooth complexion, had beautiful blue eyes that were filled with kindness and love. The three of us had a fun evening as we watched the New Year's celebration on television. Then they started counting backwards. All of a sudden Patty and Mrs. Ferguson hugged and kissed each other and me too, even though I was trying to sleep. "Happy New Year" was said over and over. Humans sure do some strange things sometimes and I still cannot understand the purpose of noisemakers. Oh, well, they are creatures of habit.

The next day was the first time I saw for myself what this panic did when it completely overcame Patty. Everything was fine when she suddenly put her hand to her chest. Then she became flushed, sweaty-looking and started breathing fast. It was like she couldn't find a place where she was comfortable. She sat down. Then she would get up and she paced. "It is happening," she told me. "Oh, Scruffy, I am so scared," she said. Unlike other attacks where they would leave, this one either was continuous or left for such a little time then started again.

She said she felt like she was going to die. She called Flo and Leonard because she didn't want to die and not be found for awhile. They came over. When they saw the condition Patty was in and how the panic attacks were continuously coming, they suggested she go home with them for a while. Patty was very passive, power-less and felt let down that she no longer was secure in her safe place, so she agreed.

We ended up staying at Flo and Leonard's house for two months. Patty had hit rock bottom. There was nowhere to go now except up that mountain. I was very happy when Flo and Leonard brought her back from an appointment with Dr. Lagoutaris. He said it was very important for Patty to go home and stay there again. She had to start facing her fears instead of avoiding them. She was missing life and I wondered why death scared her because she was not living. Flo and Leonard were great to me while we were there. I had lots of fun and went for rides in the car with Leonard. Now we had to go home—it was time.

CHAPTER FIVE

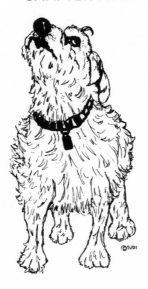

The time had come to throw myself into my mission. It was one on one now, just Patty and me. We were home, but we were spending lots of time in Patty's upstairs bedroom. It looked to me as if this was going to be her new safe place if I didn't take matters into my paws soon. Well, this should be simple enough. After all, I do have to go outside to do what dogs do, relieve myself. Also, I would like to see what is going on outside. How can I see what is going on out there from in here with all the windows shielded with closed drapes and afghans?

I had to start getting Patty's attention when I first felt the urge because I found out it took a while before we could get down the fifteen steps. Patty would make it to the top of the stairs. Then she would sit down. I sat two steps below her at all times.

I wanted to give her time to feel safe. Then I would tug at her sock, being careful so I did not bite her toes, to get her to go down one more step. Then I let her rest before I repeated the process until we finally made it to the bottom of the steps. Sometimes it went smoothly. Then there were times Patty would return to the top of the stairs and I would have to start all over. That was very frustrating to me, but I would remember that patience is a virtue. I can handle this I would tell myself. Sometimes my urge started getting more urgent.

Once we finally reached the bottom step we just had to walk across the kitchen to the back door. Patty would open the door and never stepped or looked outside but stooped to pick up my chain and attach it to my collar. I would sit there until my chain was on and then she would open the screen door. After going through this big ritual, I walked outside and relieved myself as soon as I cleared the patio. Afterwards I would sit for a while on the patio looking at the closed door. It is so hard to believe that Patty's whole world is behind that door. The world is so big. God created so much to see and do in this beautiful world. Right now my mission seems as big as the world. God help me to help her.

I had learned how to master getting my master downstairs. It was time for the next step. If I couldn't get Patty outside yet,

I would let the outside come in to her. I would sit on the back of the couch just looking at her. I would bark once, wait, and bark again. Sometimes I would whine under my breath to get her to open the drapes. At first it was one window and just a few inches of an opening of the draperies. Well, my back was getting pretty cramped because I was all hunched up trying to see things through such a small opening. After she felt safe with the draperies being opened, I would do my soft cries under my breath and give her my "sad eye" look. The opening became wider and wider until they were opened as far as they could be. Well, this is great! Now I'll do the same thing at the other end of the couch. There is a window there, too, and I will have a different view. I can see that I will have to have lots of patience to help her deal with this. Patty needs the determination to fight this. Only she can do this.

I was feeling a little mischievous. I wanted Patty to go outside if even for a few minutes. I wanted her to smell the fresh air. I wanted her to feel the air that was cold and crisp. I wanted her to hear the sounds of outside. I wanted her to see what she had been missing and have a taste of what it would be like to be free again from the solitary confinement of her house. I wanted her to experience all these things if only for a short while. One Sunday night I sat at the door as I always did to be let out. Once Patty had hooked me to the chain outside, I managed to slip out of my collar to free myself. I know I should not have done this. I was taking a big chance. Who knows, maybe Patty didn't even love me enough yet to look for me. Nah, I'll try it. I bolted through the backyard and around the house. Patty frantically screamed out, "Come back, Scruffy—Scruffy—Scruffy, OH, PLEASE COME BACK!" I was out of her sight, and she didn't know I was hiding and could see her. She was crying, but outside on the patio.

She went back into the house leaving the back door open. She opened the front door and called, "Scruffy."

Now what do I do? I thought she would run after me. She is going to the telephone. Who is she calling? Flo and Leonard are in Florida. I hear Patty say, "Gary, Scruffy just ran away. What do you mean I better go after her? I don't go outside. I don't know if I can go outside let alone go searching up and down the neighborhood. How will she know where she lives? Oh, Gary, what if she is gone? Okay, I'll do it, and I will be watching for you and Linny. Thank you, Gary." Patty thought of Gary as the brother that she never had, so it did not surprise me she turned to him. Gary was a very thoughtful and caring human. I knew this because he would do anything he could to help—deliver groceries, take Patty to see Dr. Lagoutaris or even shampoo carpets. No wonder Linny married Gary. He sure is special.

Patty came out the back door again. She started running around the house and up the center of the street yelling my name. I had never seen her move so fast. She ran one block, then two, before I knew it, three blocks, crying out my name the whole way. She stopped, I think realizing how far away she was from her home, her safe place. It wasn't like Linny and Gary could miss her. She was in the middle of the street, and her frantic cries would have led anyone to her. The whole neighborhood in fact was probably wondering who this human was. She hurriedly turned and walked as fast as she could back home!

I guess I better not carry this too far. She is coming in the front door. "Arf" I barked once but loud enough so she could hear me. She came to the back door and I stared up at her cocking my head to one side, because I know that always gets to her. Patty looked like she had seen a ghost—her eyes bigger than I had ever seen. Then, I let out another arf to snap her out of it. "Scruffy," she said with tears streaming down her face, "how did you find your way home? Please don't ever run away again. I love you."

She loves me. I knew it would happen. The bond between us was finally there. She gave me so many kisses and hugs even while she called Gary to tell him I was back.

This proved to me she could go outside and even up the street. The biggest miracle of this whole experience was she didn't have a panic attack. I came to the conclusion that in this case there was no time to think. Her first thought was of me. A human who suffers from panic attacks THINKS TOO MUCH. The two words they think of most are WHAT-IF.

Patty was always saying WHAT-IF this happens, WHAT-IF that happens. There was no doubt in my mind if she changed her self-talk, she would be on her way to living life again

CHAPTER SIX

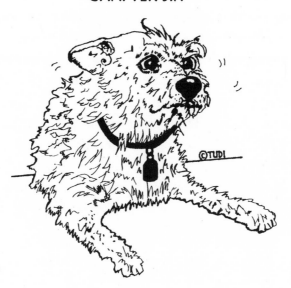

I cannot take all the credit for helping Patty with her recovery. It was truly a group effort. I had a lot of help. Patty was continuing to see Dr. Lagoutaris. He had so much faith that she could deal with this panic disorder. I hoped his faith would eventually rub off on her.

When we had come home after our two-month stay at Flo's and Leonard's, panic was not her only problem. Patty was also very depressed again. She had a feeling of hopelessness. Even though suicide was not on her mind as much anymore, there were other signs. A poor appetite or overeating is one symptom. Well, just looking at Patty we knew she did not have a poor appetite. Sometimes humans can't sleep, but Patty was sleeping too much, because I think she did not want to think about what was happening to her. Then, of course, how much can a human do in their house twenty-four hours a day; seven days a week; month after month; year after year? I also think she thought that if she slept she had less of a chance of having a panic attack. I don't think I have to mention Patty had no self-esteem; in fact, she was her own worst critic. She also had difficulty making decisions even as simple as should she pay her bills today or write a letter; and poor concentration once she did decide, to the point of not being able to write out the checks or tearing up the letter.

She didn't watch television, read or do crafts anymore all things she enjoyed doing before. Dr. Lagoutaris told her to start watching soap operas on television.

An amazing thing happened when she did this. First of all, she would be up and she got so involved she started showing emotions because of the characters on these shows. She would get angry, happy, and sad. Patty was starting to feel again and starting to express her feelings. Now this was not that easy on me. I would usually sit beside her because I do like to cuddle. Well, when she was happy she would pick me up, hold me and say, "Isn't that wonderful?" Anger would make her pick me up and yell, "Do you believe they did that, Scruffy? How can people be so conniving and devious?" When sad, she would hold me and give me a kiss on top of my head as I licked the tears from her face. Emotions are a funny thing with humans. They act a little bent out of shape when they are getting them out, but they can drive a human crazy if they don't get them out and express them.

Dr. Lagoutaris knew Patty had been an avid reader before. So, to get her started reading again, he told her to read the tabloids. He knew the articles, even with some being a little far out, would hold her interest because they were short. Some of the articles had very positive thinking ideas in them. Once again he was right. Patty read an article; then a page; a couple of pages, until she finished the whole thing. Then she went to books. The first book she read was *Living, Loving & Learning* by Leo Buscaglia, Ph.D. given to her by Flo.

Patty was reading *Living, Loving & Learning* and within the first ten pages she read something that had a very big impact on her. Dr. Buscaglia relates the story of a girl. A student who was "absolutely brilliant, whose mind was exciting, who had creativity like you never dreamed" that had committed suicide.[1]

This experience had such a big impact on Dr. Buscaglia and after reading his book, *Love*, Patty found out that was the reason he started his Love class at the University of Southern California. [2]

In ending the book *Living, Loving & Learning* Dr. Buscaglia says:

47

"To hope is to risk pain." And, "To try is to risk failure. But risk must be taken, because the greatest hazard in life is to risk nothing. The person who risks nothing does nothing, has nothing, and is nothing. He may avoid suffering and sorrow, but he simply cannot learn, feel, change, grow, live, or love. Chained by his certitudes or his addictions, he's a slave. He has forfeited his greatest trait, and that is his individual freedom. Only the person who risks is free.

"To keep you hidden, to lose you because of self-defeating ideas is to die. Don't let that happen. Your greatest responsibility is to become everything that you are, not only for your benefit, but for mine." [3]

Even though Patty had never even heard of Leo Buscaglia, he had helped her realize suicide was not the answer. Finding her self-esteem was. He would sometimes be on the Public Broadcasting station where he once said you should even love your fat thighs, which made her laugh. Her thighs were not what she was concerned about. Patty was in size eighteen maternity clothes because her weight was everywhere but her thighs. As she looked in the mirror she said to me, "Look, Scruffy, I have no neck. It looks like my jaws go right into my shoulders." She laughed and went on to say she once heard inside every thin Taurus there is a fat one trying to get out. "Well, Scruffy, look at me. I have doubled my weight. Where did this other person come from?"

Dr. Lagoutaris had told Patty that sometimes when you are on medication one of the side effects could be weight gain. They both were very honest with each other that eating habits were also a factor here. Patty decided to start being much more aware of anything she put in her mouth. Dr. Lagoutaris also told her that he thought it was important to exercise. One of the benefits of exercise was that natural chemicals called endorphins are released. When released, these endorphins help calm a person, help generate positive energy and are great stress regulators. Patty realized exercise would not only help her mental outlook, but also help her lose weight. This would also give her a feeling of accomplishment, which would help her self-esteem. It would also help save the furniture. After all she had already broken one couch with a queen size bed in it.

Patty had an exercise bike that had gone unused. At first she was lucky if she could go half of a mile. Some days she got on the bike twice to reach that half a mile. Gradually she worked her way up to five miles a day, then five miles twice a day. Around this time a friend of hers from Florida came to visit. A licensed aerobics instructor who worked out an exercise program with weights for her to do at home.

Patty recalled what Dr. Lagoutaris had told her about the mountain. Recovery is like climbing a mountain. You keep climbing and sometimes you slide back down a little, but you just keep on climbing and you'll reach your castle at the top. Patty had started her climb. At some time during this climb she was going to have to attack her panic. I felt pawsitive she would do it.

One day Patty was reading the newspaper and said, "Scruffy, will you look at this? There is a behavior modification group starting to help agoraphobic and panic sufferers. It says that this course will help with phobias." She said, "I have never seen anything like this before." I could tell she was excited because I was getting so many kisses and hugs, I'm sure the curl on top of my head was flat now. "This program sounds like it really could help me deal with what I have." Then she stopped.

"How can I even do this? I have not driven or been with any strangers for five years now." She called the telephone number and asked that more information be sent.

When she had her next appointment with Dr. Lagoutaris, she took the information with her. They decided to start phone counseling with this counselor first. She would then start individual counseling and when the next group started in six months or so, Patty would be more prepared. When the time had finally come, Flo picked her up to take her to her first two-hour session. Patty was told she could bring a support person with her if she wanted. However, Patty chose not to, thinking she would then probably have to go to another group to learn how to let go of the support person. No, she decided to do this on her own. I was proud of her, even though she doesn't realize I am her Support Dog.

At her first session she told me she met nine other people who suffered from panic disorder and half had panic disorder with agoraphobia. Patty knew how severe her case was when she listened to the others relate their stories. One lady there only had panic attacks when she turned left in traffic. She felt she had the most work to do. Patty was told the more she put into the course the more she would benefit. She knew that only she could solve her own problem. During this first session Patty learned to rate her symptoms on a scale from one to ten. She was told it was very important to be aware of her symptoms as she practiced. As she listened and followed along in her manual she cold hardly wait to ATTACK THIS PANIC instead of letting the PANIC ATTACK HER.

TABLE 1 - THE ANXIETY SCALE

AREA OF NON-FUNCTION

10. Panic: disoriented, spacey, detached, frantic, hysterical numbness, or weird sensations and feelings

9. Dizziness, nausea, diarrhea, visual distortion, numbness, some hysterical sensations, concern for losing control

8. Stiff neck, headache, feeling of doom

AREA OF DECREASED ABILITY TO FUNCTION

7. Tight chest, hyperventilation

6. Lump in throat, strong muscle tension

5. Dry mouth, feelings of need for escape, or hide

4. Shaky legs, feel wobbly

AREA OF CONTINUED ABILITY TO FUNCTION

3. Rapid or strong heartbeat, tremor, muscle tension

2. Sweaty or clammy palms, warm all over

1. Butterflies in stomach

Adapted from Terrap Self-Help Program by Arthur B. Hardy, M.D. (USA: TSC Management Corp., 1981), III, p. 6.

The counselor who was in charge of the behavior modification had two helpers. One of these helpers was a recovering agoraphobic with whom Patty felt an immediate bond with because she thought if this woman could do it so can she. At that first group meeting, she learned they would be using a desensitization method, that there would be homework each week, and lots of practice—LOTS OF PRACTICE.

When Flo brought Patty home that day, she was overwhelmed with all she had learned in two hours. It was almost overpowering considering all she had to do to recover. She decided not to look at it like that, but as a step at a time—a step up her mountain. Only she could do it. She said, "Scruffy, I have so much work to do to get better, but I have started."

When practicing and using the desensitization method you must first be relaxed. So Patty would do her relaxation exercises and visualize what she was going to attempt to do. She always gave herself permission to retreat if her anxiety level was starting to go into panic.

The first thing she did was to go out on her back patio. Even though it was cold she would stay out a little longer each time. Patty kept Mrs. Ferguson informed on what she was doing. That Mrs. Ferguson was something else! The one window of her apartment, when opened up gave her a view of Patty's back patio. Whenever she knew Patty was out there she would open it up and they would talk.

On the first day of spring, the telephone rang and it was Mrs. Ferguson. After Patty got off the telephone she said that Mrs. Ferguson had told her to come to the "drive-thru window" on the patio. When Patty opened the door even I couldn't believe it. There were all different colored flags decorating the window. Mrs. Ferguson first directed Patty to pick a number from a basket to see if she had won the door prize of the Grand Opening of the Drive-Thru-Window. Naturally she had, and Mrs. Ferguson gave her a gift. She passed out a dinner plate and believe me it smelled good. Mrs. Ferguson is one really special female human and I knew she had hit on something because Patty would be out on that patio, especially if food was involved.

The next thing we did was go and sit on Mrs. Ferguson's screened-in porch. So what if her apartment was attached to the house, we were still sitting outside. It was great to be in the fresh air. I felt like one lucky dog. I had hit the jackpot because her porch had a great corner view and I could see so much compared to the windows in our living room, which at least were no longer covered by afghans.

I also got to meet two lovely female humans, who joined us on the porch. Marion and Anna Mae were sisters who lived on the other side of Mrs. Ferguson. I didn't even know I had neighbors other than Mrs. Ferguson. I listened as Patty told these three friendly humans about her behavior modification group. They were so excited and willingly offered to help in any way they could since they had the time, now that they were retired. It was decided right then and there that after Patty got home from her group sessions the four of them would get together to discuss what she had learned. Then they would help her with her homework for the next week. Most of all, these humans were giving her a lot of encouragement and love. Marion and Anna Mae both told Patty, "Pretty soon you will be able to come and sit on our porch." I looked over to their porch and there were three sides I could look out from there. Reality set in. It was sixteen yards to their porch. It was so close, but yet so far away in Patty's mind. "Someday," she said, "someday."

I was really proud of Patty. Each time Flo would bring her home from yet another group session I could see how much more determined she was. She would repeat Dr. Lagoutaris's words and say, "Scruffy, I am climbing to the top of the mountain to my castle. I might slide down a bit, but I will get to that castle." She would listen to her relaxation tapes. She would visualize herself going places and doing things again. She would see herself in control.

I would never minimize anything that Patty worked on because each step she took was a big one. She would be exhausted after trying each new experience. After all, she was learning one of the biggest lessons in life—how to live again.

"The car, Scruffy," she said one day, "it is time."

I was really excited jumping up and down; wagging my tail because I just loved to go for rides. What views I can see from a car! Patty had already started her thought process before she even said this. She knew that the car was in good working order even though she had not driven for years. There was a male human named Bill who had kept the car in good condition for her. He would take it for inspections and make repairs that had to be done. I really liked Bill. I knew he was a real animal lover because of the stories he told about his dog, Dudley. Anyone who loves animals has a big, gentle, kind heart in my book. Bill was also one of the humans who came over to see us while we were in the house. He would bring us some really good chicken and always made Patty laugh. I know being the sensitive human he was, he could not understand what had happened to her because he had known her before when she was active, but he didn't question her.

One time, Patty and I were sitting on the patio and he not only brought the car back but also his brother, Vern, who was visiting from Oklahoma. After they had left Patty said, "Scruffy, that Vern seemed really nice, too bad he lives in Oklahoma."

After we listened to a relaxation tape, Patty went to the door with keys in hand. She sat on the patio for a few minutes. She rose and walked up the driveway until she reached the car. She unlocked it. Then she got in and rolled down the window. There she sat for five minutes like a child human turning the wheel, visualizing herself driving. I couldn't believe it; I was ready for a ride and it was over before the car even started. The next time she sat in the car longer and on it went until one day SHE STARTED THE CAR. I could not believe my eyes when I saw the car MOVE. Okay, so she was just driving up and down the driveway, but she was DRIVING. She was so excited as she came over to me on the patio, hugging me, kissing the top of my head, smashing my curl screaming, "Scruffy, I DID IT—I DID IT. I AM SO EXCITED." Well, there was no stopping her after that. Next I went for a ride with her. So it was just around the block. To us it felt like we had gone five hundred miles. Patty kept on practicing until she felt comfortable.

Patty called Flo one day before her group meeting and said she would appreciate it if Flo would follow her while she drove her own car. I knew Flo would be surprised and very happy to agree. She told Patty she would return after the group was over so she could follow Patty home. Soon after, she drove all by herself knowing she could call if it was necessary. A total of 4.3 miles, but that was far towards Patty's road to recovery. Talk about kisses and hugs! No dog could have had more than the day she drove without having Flo follow her. "I DID IT, SCRUFFY, I DROVE ALL BY MYSELF!" This was one of these moments when humans cry because they are happy. I shed a couple of tears myself as I licked Patty's tears from her face.

I don't want to give you the impression that everything Patty tried went smoothly. One time, I remember she was an hour late coming home from group therapy. I was concerned as I looked out the window. This was not like Patty. I knew she would not have gone shopping. When she got home she looked more exhausted than I had ever seen her. She said, "Scruffy, I had a full-blown panic attack during group. We were doing a desensitization exercise looking at pictures. There was a picture of an airplane. I lost it. My counselor would not let me come home until she was sure I was alright." This was the first time she had a panic attack at group. She did not let it stop her though.

As the "I CAN'T DO IT" became "I CAN DO IT," I could see Patty continuing to grow. The group took field trips, after which Patty always came home to tell the female humans and me on Mrs. Ferguson's porch all that happened. There was always anticipation before she went on one of these field trips. She was learning to decipher the difference between anxiety, panic, anticipation, and excitement. On this particular day, Patty had gone to a department store that seemed to be an acre in size. She related that the group traveled together. The counselor and two leaders each had three phobic humans for more individual help if needed. The suggestion was to wear sunglasses in the store because, for some reason unknown to me, fluorescent lighting can have a strange effect on humans.

Patty laughed as she told the story to the now "Porch Club" saying, "We looked like a group who was disguising our identity." I must say, Patty never lost her sense of humor through this whole thing.

"I have to laugh," she would say, "without humor this would be so very depressing."

When going shopping, they could stay around the front of the store but they had to buy one thing. Sometimes, the TV Guide at the checkout counter seemed too far back from the entrance to the store. Each trip would take her farther into the store.

The day the group went on a field trip to the mall, Patty came home not only excited over her accomplishment, but while she was there she had a second hole pierced into her ears. She said, "I have always wanted to have this done, but now I will never forget the significance of this day."

CHAPTER SEVEN

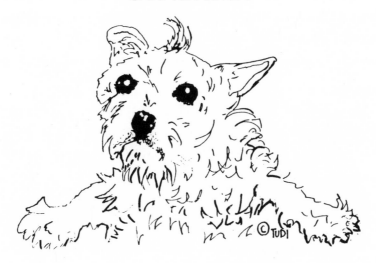

The behavior modification course continued for almost a year in human time. Faithfully, Patty was there each time the group met. Physical exercise, mental relaxation exercises, homework, and practicing became a daily way of life for her. She realized there were two things that could be done with this panic disorder. You could let it control you as she had done, or take charge of yourself physically and mentally to control the panic.

Patty learned that when a panic attack started you should not start the WHAT-IF thinking. A human can actually make a panic attack last longer by doing this. Instead she learned ways to divert her thinking.

A rubber band worn around her wrist was one. The purpose of the rubber band was to snap it to bring yourself to the present when you started to think WHAT- IF.

Breathing is one of the most important things she learned. She became very aware of how she breathed especially during a panic attack. Breathing in calmness EVER SO SLOWLY through her nose; exhaling anxiety EVER SO SLOWLY through her mouth so that if she had a lit candle in front of her the flame would not go out.

Something so simple as the alphabet was another excellent diversion. You simply go through the alphabet thinking of three-letter words. If you are still experiencing panic or anxiety you continue with four-letter words and so on.

Patty laughed when she told me about these diversions saying, "Scruffy, I would have paid anything to be able to control panic and really it does not cost anything, unless you have to buy rubber bands."

Patty became a good friend with Vicki, one of the leaders of the group. Vicki became Patty's role model because she herself had been through this course, and now she was a recovering agoraphobic in control enough to help others. Vicki was the example that it could be done. Vicki introduced a valuable tool to the thought process of recovery with Patty—audiotapes. The first tape that Vicki shared with her was one by Zig Ziglar. On this particular tape he said a person has to get rid of their STINKING THINKING. This one audiotape had a big impact on Patty and paved the way to a new way of thinking. Patty would be exercising and say, "Look, Scruffy, I am getting rid of my STINKING THINKING," or she would be doing her practicing and say laughingly, "Scruffy, I am getting rid of my STINKING THINKING." Yes, I heard a lot about STINKING THINKING; in fact she would even ask me if I was getting rid of my STINKING THINKING. I could not believe these two words could have had such an impact on her. Of course these two words were better than WHAT-IF.

Anthony Robbins, Wayne Dwyer, and Robert Schuller also had made very motivating, positive audio tapes that Vicki shared with Patty. These tapes unlocked her old negative thinking process so that it could be replaced with positive thoughts. Patty was familiar with positive thinking because every Sunday she would watch The *Hour of Power* with Dr. Robert Schuller. Also, she had read *The Power of Positive Thinking* by Norman Vincent Peale. She had no idea how much more information there was about the subject.

Positive thinking and visualization were both fairly new to her since everything in the world seemed so negative. Patty listened to every tape and read every article and book that she could on the subjects. Her conquest over panic was like conquering the enemy. This was not a battle to her. It was a war. Individual counseling sessions with Dr. Lagoutaris, behavior modification, exercising, practicing positive thinking, and visualization were her weapons. All of the above were helping her climb her mountain. She was doing it slowly—one step at a time.

Patty also learned the importance of remembering to ALWAYS give yourself permission to retreat. Even more importantly, NOT TO BE CRITICAL of yourself, if you do retreat. There is always the next time. Always give yourself CREDIT for each step you take. Also PRAISE YOURSELF. Concentrate on positive things about the qualities you possess.

Be open about your panic disorder. There is nothing to be ashamed of, so don't try to hide it. Over three million humans suffer from panic disorder. You are not alone because it is, at present, the number one mental disorder. Think of it as having the most popular disorder. You are in style.

When Patty first experienced these feelings and didn't know what she had, there was nothing much about it on television. Then Oprah Winfrey did a show on agoraphobia. There was also a soap opera called *Capitol* in which one of the characters supposedly was suffering from agoraphobia. Now, every talk show and even news programs such as *20-20* have featured information about this disorder.

No one knows why Panic Disorder happens. There are many opinions. Whatever the reason you suffer from it, doing something about it is the answer. Knowing you can live with panic disorder should help you. Even humans who do not have a panic disorder get panicky for some reason or another. The things that make them panicky are called phobias. I will be perfectly honest with you, I have a few myself—brontophobia, fear of thunder. Other things that make me panicky are balloons, squeak toys, and firecrackers, and I dread the Fourth of July. I put a list of over one hundred phobias[1] in the back of my book to calm your fears that you are not alone.

Look at the positive side. You DO NOT DIE from panic disorder. I think that speaks for itself.

You will feel a great SENSE OF ACCOMPLISHMENT when you start controlling the panic instead of it controlling you. Then, if you are also agoraphobic like Patty and never leave your house, you save money on clothes. You never seem to wear out your shoes. You save money on gasoline and wear and tear on tires. A tank of gas lasted for years because Bill put on the only miles that were on Patty's car.

Of course, you are missing your most precious gift which is living life. I can remember one time Patty saying to me, "I have come so far, Scruffy; however, will I ever see the things I miss so much?"

Mickey Mouse — oh, yes, Patty was a real Mickey Mouse fan. The ocean, plays, live concerts, and traveling were some of the things she longed to have back in her life. Patty told me about the time when she was watching Diana Ross doing a live concert on television in Central Park. Diana was going to sing *Reach Out and Touch Someone*, and told everyone in the audience to hold hands while she sang this song. Patty placed her hand on the television set as she sang along with Diana.

Thank goodness that all the new cable-shopping channels which are now on television were not on during this time of Patty's confinement. There seemed to be another frequent male human who stopped at our house during this period. Patty called him the UPS man. Patty would see something on television and order it. I think this happened because all humans shop and I think she missed shopping, or she wanted to remain knowledgeable about new products that were available now. I remember this one item she ordered, a portable dishwasher for $19.95. I know it sure did make her laugh when it came. The portable dishwasher turned out to be a little brush that screwed onto the faucet, and when the water was turned on its force made the brush spin.

"Oh, Scruffy, it is portable," she said, "but I have to go shopping myself to see what I am purchasing."

Patty was driving to and from her group and therapy sessions. There was another way she continued improving. Our friend, Bill, had an auto body business and when Bill had to take a car back to someone, or pick one up, Patty would follow him. A few times they stopped for a bite to eat and this was the start of Patty going back into restaurants. Patty would tell me that Bill would talk about his girlfriend, Carol, who Patty didn't know. She thought how nice it would be to be in a relationship. She wondered if she would ever date again. Her world was still so small, how would she meet someone?

"Maybe a repairman," or she would laugh and say, "did you ever notice a wedding ring on the UPS man, Scruffy?" Then, more seriously, she would say, "Most of all how could anyone understand what I am battling?"

Patty was now feeling more secure driving and on this particular day announced, "Scruffy, you have an appointment with Dr. Baker for your checkup and I am going to take you."

I always liked seeing Dr. Baker and the girls at the office, but until this time it was always Flo or Leonard who took me for my checkups. I would always give Dr. Baker lots of kisses and be really excited to see him. I have heard of other dogs that might just have a little phobia of their own because when they go to the doctor's, they shake, cry and don't want to get out of the car. Not me, and certainly not today. I was very happy Dr. Baker was finally going to meet my Master. I knew he would be proud of me because I had been such a good Support Dog. He would know that I had been working on my mission.

Patty was not only taking care of my needs, she was starting to take care of her own as well. Patty had known a dentist named Dr. Fridley, who limited his practice to Periodontics and

Oral Diagnosis. Leonard had been the athletic team doctor for years at a local high school. When Patty was very young Leonard would take her and Linny with him when he attended to the athletes. Dr. Fridley at that time was on the basketball team, and he seemed so very tall to Patty. He could not have seemed taller in her eyes; however, when she explained her panic disorder to him, he understood. She was very honest about what her feelings were when the panic occurred. Lightheadedness, nausea, chest pains, and the urgency to flee if she felt threatened were all reasons she had not kept up her regular six-month checkup with her dentist. The years of not being able to go to the dentist had left a lot of work to be done. Also, certain medications and poor eating habits caused her teeth to be discolored. When Patty smiled, she smiled crookedly because she was so self-conscious about her teeth. Because she previously had beautiful teeth, this really bothered her. She told him about her therapy, her behavior modification, and that which she had learned about positive thinking and visualization, which he thought were all very important and things he believed in very much.

Dr. Fridley explained that as she continued to work on her panic disorder and became able to decrease her medication, much more could be done to correct her dental problems. The process to do this would involve a lot of appointments with his colleague, Dr. Generalovich, whom Patty didn't know. She would have to prepare herself mentally but the results would be her dream come true. She came home and told me about what Dr. Fridley had said. "I have to learn to control this panic more to be able to cut down on my medication, Scruffy." She went on, "This will be my graduation present to myself because I plan on smiling a lot when I am in control."

She learned that desensitization could also be used when going to a doctor's office. She also learned to visit the doctor's office to make her appointment instead of calling. This process only took a few minutes, but she had a visual picture of the office. She also knew where she was going and met some of the office staff, explaining to them that she had panic disorder. Asking to be the first patient of the day so she did not have all day to think about her appointment. She would be seen first and did not have to wait long because other patients were ahead of her. I also have some tips myself to add that might help. Take someone with you for support. Also, know that by the same time tomorrow it will be over and that this time next year you will most likely not even remember you had an appointment.

CHAPTER EIGHT

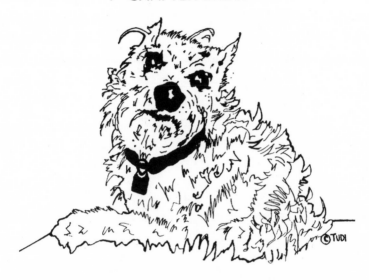

Patty graduated on February 13, 1986, from her behavior modification class. She continued with her individual counseling and her sessions with Dr. Lagoutaris. When she had come home after a session with Dr. Lagoutaris, she said, "Scruffy, Dr. Lagoutaris is so happy with my progress. He is pleased that I am continuing to exercise not only physically, but mentally exercising what I have learned with my positive thinking, visualization and practicing to go a little further with things I was avoiding. Remember Scruffy, when the only way I could get my hair done was if Livie came here to do it? I told him I found a small beauty shop that I go to and I feel comfortable. My next step will be going to the larger beauty shop where Livie works.

"I told Dr. Lagoutaris that to reach my castle at the top of the mountain seems to be taking forever. He said that it had taken years for me to get the way I was, so why did I think changing my thinking should be instantaneous. It takes time, but he said, 'Once you're at the top you will never allow yourself to slide down to the bottom again. At times in your life you might slide down a little, but you will catch yourself before you slide too far.' Damn it, Scruffy, I've come too far to stop now."

I want to tell you from experience that when Patty says, "damn it," she is mad. I know humans say only dogs get mad but when Patty says that, I KNOW she is mad. I knew she was not mad at me. She was mad at the way the panic had taken over her whole life for so many years. Even though she had progressed a great deal, she still had to be one step ahead of it. She had to change her whole self-talk and thought processes and learn how to live life over again. She was doing well.

Dr. Lagoutaris suggested that it was time for her to start doing volunteer work. This would get her out a few hours each week. Volunteering not only benefits the organization you volunteer for, but humans get a lot of self-satisfaction.

Patty talked to her female human friend, Margie, about what Dr. Lagoutaris had said about volunteering. Margie, who had majored in Health and Physical Education, had helped Patty a lot and was a positive influence, suggesting healthier eating habits and more home exercising. Patty was now out of her size eighteen maternity clothes and had thirty more pounds to lose to reach her desired weight. I enjoyed the fact that Patty was eating healthier because that meant I was also eating healthier. Since Patty still could not go for walks, I had to watch my weight. With my frame I have to stick close to fifteen pounds, never going over seventeen pounds. Gosh, when Patty started exercising and eating healthier, she had to lose half of herself. Even though I did not get to go for walks I was getting my exercise. Patty was now able to open the front door of our house. There was a love seat positioned in front of that door. I would continuously be jumping to the back of the love seat so I could see what was happening in the neighborhood. Believe me I would bark if some strange dog looked like he was getting too close to my territory. I would also bark if strange humans came too close to the house. I also greeted the humans that came to visit. I was one busy dog. My list of duties other than being supportive was endless. Patty would call me Mrs. Kravitz, who was a character in *Bewitched*, a television show that had a nosy neighbor. I didn't care. I was so happy to have the doors opened.

Patty and Margie decided to volunteer at the F. H. Buhl Club. The Buhl Club was a gift to the Shenango Valley, in 1903, by philanthropist Frank H. Buhl. The club had been very influential in molding positive characteristics of children in the area for years. The club had activities that included lessons in dance, gymnastics, swimming, and martial arts. It had programs for preschool and game rooms for the teenagers. Adults were not excluded for there was a variety of exercise programs with many different rooms and specific exercise equipment.

So not only would Patty volunteer, but she would also familiarize herself with the club and eventually feel comfortable in reaping the benefits of exercising there.

Carolyn Williams was in charge of the volunteer program. She was also the Director of Special Activities.

Patty explained her panic disorder and Carolyn was very considerate with placing Patty. She told her if she ever felt the need to leave to let her know. They talked about where Patty would feel the safest. Because of her love for children, it was decided she would help with the baby- sitting program. Margie also volunteered for baby-sitting the same day and time as Patty. This arrangement made Patty feel very secure.

She met so many wonderful humans there — Tony, the Director; Barb, the secretary; and Peggy, the supervisor were just a few. Everything she told me about them upheld the feeling that her choice had been a good one. These humans were caring, considerate, and thoughtful. "It is like being a part of a family," she would tell me, "my club family."

The next year when it was time to volunteer, Patty was in charge of the baby-sitting program. Next she worked the front desk. I sure wish we dogs had clubs where we could go. I know there is a Kennel Club, but I hear it is hard to become a member.

Not only did Patty develop a love for these humans, but also a miracle happened. Patty loved people her whole life, but she thought that if she loved herself she would be selfish. She could not understand how humans could say you have to love yourself first before you love anyone else.

During her appointment with Dr. Lagoutaris, in April of 1987, Patty told him, "At the age of thirty-eight, I have finally found THE GREATEST LOVE OF ALL. I now truly know what it's like to love myself. I have developed such a great sense of SELF-ESTEEM. Only I can make myself happy, no one else. I realize I have been my toughest critic. I have been so hard on myself. I have accomplished so very much and I am so excited. I am so proud of myself. I know my castle is now within reach."

Patty's new attitude made me very happy. It was like a big weight had been lifted from her shoulders. She was fun before, but now she was even more fun. Sometimes even a little silly— like the night we were watching television and she held me. Looking at me she said, "Scruffy, I have something to tell you, I think you are old enough to handle this. I am not your natural mother. You were adopted but I have loved you like you were my own."

What she didn't know was I had adopted her as my mission.

Humans are not the only ones that need a little help with their assignments in life. The time had come when I needed a little help here. It seemed I had done all I could think of to help Patty. She never stopped practicing, but our world was still very limited. There were times when I wanted to throw my paws up in the air because I didn't know how to get Patty to go further. I know I am not the only one who feels this way. Even all the humans who have helped don't know what the next step should be. I asked my Boss, the Creator, for help. I told Him I felt I had done a good job. I also told Him I felt Patty was really doing a good job. I told Him I felt she was at a standstill and I asked Him for help. Christmas was coming and it always brings miracles. It would also be my third anniversary with Patty. I know, Creator, You hear me. You tell humans to ask and they shall receive. I know You also hold Your animals in a very special place. You even gave them their own saint, St. Francis. His feast day is in October and Patty took me to church where they have a ceremony to bless the animals. There were all kinds of pets there—hamsters, gerbils, rabbits, goldfish, cats and of course, doggies. Tudi is visiting today because she and Patty are going to the Humane Society to look for a dog to adopt for Flo.

Just then, there was a knock at the back door. Oh good, it is our friend, Bill, bringing Patty's car back from being inspected. He has someone with him. He was tall and looked like he took exercising as seriously as we do. His brown hair covered his forehead and he had a mustache. He was very good-looking, distinguished and had thoughtful, inquisitive eyes. I remember this male human. He is Bill's brother, Vern.

Bill and Vern came in and sat down in the living room. Bill knew Tudi, and Patty introduced Tudi to Vern. I listened as Patty and Tudi talked about going to look for a dog for Flo, and that Leonard was in on the surprise. Truthfully speaking, I was not real happy about getting a cousin. After all, I had been the main and only dog in this family's life for three years. But, on second thought, how could I not want another dog that needs a home in our family. At least I could relate to him or her in our own language. There would be no guessing what we were saying. This human family has so much love to go around. Their feelings for me will not change. I will not let them forget who was here first!

I watched and listened as Patty asked Vern if he was home for the holidays. I could not believe my big ears, so I knew I heard right when he said he had moved from Oklahoma in August and was a professor at Mercyhurst College eighty miles away. As the conversation between Vern and Patty went on, there was something I had never seen before happen with Patty. There was a look about her. She had always talked a lot with her eyes because they were very expressive. Even if she was not talking, you could tell with those blue eyes if she was happy, sad, scared, hurt, or worried. Now there was an extra sparkle that I had never seen before, a look of calmness and trust.

Dogs are sometimes penned in so they don't run away. Humans put up their own barriers, which I never could understand, so they feel protected. This Vern, however, was breaking through the wall of protection Patty had built around herself. I could tell!

When Bill and Vern left, I knew he was the quickest answer to my prayer. Sometimes you think your answer will never come. This answer arrived special delivery. I could tell Vern was special.

Christmas and New Year's came and went. Patty was not even a little let down or sad when it was over. My human really loves Christmas. How much does she love Christmas? Well, on June 25th she gets excited because Christmas is only six months away. She puts her Christmas decorations up at the beginning of November although she does wait until Thanksgiving to turn the lights on. Flo even told me that when Patty was in her first apartment and got her Christmas tree, she left the tree up until February and put Valentine decorations on it because she did not want to take it down. Then, there is this sound humans make called whistling. Patty whistles Christmas songs from November on through the holidays.

One particular day, as she took her decorations down, she said, "Scruffy, Christmas is over and it is time to move on and live. It is time to go further. It is time to stop protecting myself against people. I believe that is what I have been doing."

This was just three days into the New Year and Patty went to the telephone and called Bill. I just sat there amazed when I heard her say, "Hi, Bill, how were your holidays?" I got as close as I could to her because sometimes you can hear what the other person is saying if you get close enough. "Bill, the reason I am calling is about Vern. I know he is not married, but is he involved with anyone?"

Bill said, "No, why?"

"Because I would like to go out with him," Patty replied.

Bill shrieked, "What! But Patty, you don't date anyone. At least you haven't for eight years."

"I know I haven't but there is something about Vern. I feel that I would be safe with him, that he is very considerate and would be understanding. I would like to go out with him," Patty said.

"This is great. I think you two would be good for each other." Bill went on, "I'll be calling him because his birthday is this Thursday. I'll get back to you. Bye."

"Thank you, Bill," Patty said as she hung the telephone up. She came over and hugged me every so lightly saying, "I can't believe I did that. I have not been so spontaneous for years."

Two days later the telephone rang. "Hello," Patty said. "Bill, how are you doing? He does! He will! That will be great! Bye."

Hot dog, I thought. I knew this would work as Patty came over, picked me up, and started hugging me. "Oh, Scruffy, that was Bill. Vern wants to get together and we are going out this Saturday. Bill said he will have a bite to eat with us and then Vern and I will be on our own. Scruffy, I have a date for this Saturday—I won't be watching the *Golden Girls*," she laughed. "Do you believe it?"

"Yes, I believe it," I thought. I needed some help. I asked the Creator. He always listens. Now, please put me down. *Lassie* is on television and I really like watching her.

Saturday came and Patty had not called Bill to cancel. She was excited. "I can do this," she kept repeating to herself.

There was a knock at the back door. It was Vern. I don't know how much he knew about Patty's situation, but I had a feeling Bill had brought him up to date. He came in very confident and I sensed he felt protective of Patty. He leaned down to kiss her lightly. He really is tall I thought; at least the tallest male human I have ever seen. I tried to make him feel welcome by telling him how excited I was to see him. He bent over to pet me. I gave him a kiss and I know he really liked me because he asked Patty if he could give me a treat. He looked at Patty and said, "Are you ready to become a millionaire? The lottery jackpot is eighteen million in Ohio so let's go buy a ticket before we meet Bill. We can split our winnings. I feel very lucky tonight."

Patty made sure the front door was locked and that the television was on for me. I love watching television, especially *Lassie, Mr. Ed*, cowboy movies, and anything with a ball in it. She left the television on for me when she started leaving the house; since we were together all the time, I was happy to have some time for myself to lay back and watch some television. She also put some treats on the couch for me.

I watched as Patty and Vern walked to the back door. I watched the door close. I heard the key in the door as it re-opened. I held my breath as I heard Patty say, "I'll just be a minute. I want to make sure I unplugged my electric rollers."

I knew she had because she always puts them away after she uses them. She ran upstairs. I followed her. She stooped down and hugged me as she did a breathing exercise. "Scruffy, I will be fine." I knew that, but sometimes she says that to convince herself. "Okay, now I'm ready."

We went downstairs and Vern was at the door. I looked up at him. He knew I was entrusting my Master to him. He took Patty's hand as they left again shutting the door. I waited. I heard the car starting up. It is going down the driveway. I waited. They didn't come back. It was quite a while before I moved into the living room to watch television and eat my treats. I also thanked my Creator for answering my prayer. I know some female humans who always say they can never meet any-one no matter where they go or what they do. Then there is my

Master, Patty, who was in the house for years. She went out on her porch one day and met Vern from Oklahoma. Years later, she's out of the house and out with Vern who lives close to us now. Thank you, Creator, I could have never pulled this one off.

CHAPTER NINE

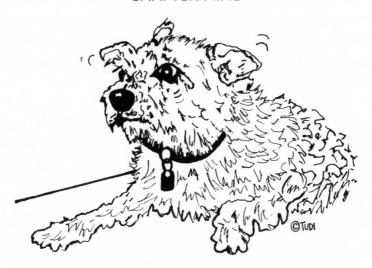

In 1988 the movie *Beaches* was released and the title song from that movie was *The Wind Beneath My Wings*. I personally always liked the song *How Much Is That Doggie In The Window?* Vern, however, became the wind beneath Patty's wings right from their first date. On that date she explained panic disorder and agoraphobia to him. Patty felt that if Vern knew about this and if ever she felt the need to go home, he would not take it personally or think she wasn't having a good time. She asked him if she could be assured he would bring her home. He reassured her that he would. "I just had to know you would, even though it might never happen," she replied. It never did.

Vern started reading articles and books on agoraphobia and panic disorder so he could help Patty. They had been dating for a month when he suggested that she come to Erie to see where he lived. He gave her a map with so many landmarks on it that I could have found where he lived. He also gave her his schedule when and where he could be reached if she needed him.

This was a big step up that mountain and I got to go, too. Finally, after all these years I got a really long ride in the car. She did not travel the interstate at first but went through small towns. By doing this, she felt she could stop if it was necessary, thus dividing the eighty miles to Erie into three smaller trips— Our home to Greenville, Greenville to Meadville and Meadville to Erie. I did not mind at all because I got to see lots of animals by going this way. We had no problems and drove right to his house.

Vern was waiting for us and we had such a good time seeing all the sights of Erie. First on our tour was Mercyhurst, the small private college where Vern taught. The huge black iron gates welcomed you to the picturesque setting of the college. The buildings combined history with continuing expansion of modern-day architecture. As our tour continued, I realized Erie was much bigger than Sharon. There was even this big lake. Vern was ready for me because I even got my own dishes to eat and drink from and a chain that was attached to his back porch so I could see what was going on in his neighborhood. He also had a couch in front of the window. This was great. I could tell he really was taken with me. When he was sitting in his recliner, I would sit next to him.

The evening before we were supposed to leave to go home, the weather human on television said there might be snow. The thought of driving in snow would cause Patty an almost certain panic attack. Vern sure was smart because he sensed what was happening.

He said, "Patty, why the worried look about the snow reports? If it snows you can stay until it melts. You could take a bus and I will get your car back to you or I could drive you home and find a way back. So, now that you don't have to worry, is there anything else you want to concern yourself over?"

They both laughed hysterically. It sure was a relief having Vern help me with this mission because he could communicate so much better with Patty. What he was telling her was that there is always at least one solution to a worry, sometimes more. Even though Patty had been working on her self-talk and positive thinking, it takes a constant effort to remember this when your thinking has been negative for so long. And humans have the nerve to say it is hard to teach an old dog new tricks!

Patty was doing things that she had not done for a long time. When Vern would sense Patty's anxiety rising he reminded her to use her rubber band, to think positively and to stop the WHAT-IFS. Vern would also tell Patty how proud he was of her when she did something that was an extra challenge to her even when she didn't say anything about being apprehensive. I told you that Vern was smart and that Patty did a lot of talking with her eyes.

One time when we were in Erie, Patty and Vern went to a very big grocery store. Patty could not believe all the new products that had come out during her years of confinement. She told Vern that people must have thought she was from an impoverished foreign country. There is another observation I have made about Patty. When she is very excited about something her whole body gets excited; you can tell by looking at her that she is excited. There she is in this huge grocery store, proclaiming her amazement about all of the new "Rice-a-Roni" products, the noodles, reduced-calorie food, Chinese and Mexican sections in the freezers. If someone was beside her, she would say to them, "Do you believe all these products that have come out?" As they looked at her in disbelief. It was a whole new world in the grocery store.

Patty's friend, Terry, had moved to Virginia Beach from Pittsburgh and Patty really wanted to see her and the ocean. Vern knew this and during our first summer together, he took Patty to Virginia Beach. As she sat on the shore looking out at the ocean, tears streamed down her face and it was the longest time before she could even speak. "Thank you so very much, Vern, for bringing me to see Terry and the ocean. Life is more beautiful than I remember it being."

Her senses were keener than ever. Maybe she took them for granted.

She saw things she had never seen before—the mood of the ocean as the waves rolled into the shore; the sea gulls hovering over the water and flying to the rocks to rest before flying off again; how the sky and the ocean created the illusion that they met; how the tides stroked the sand on the beach; and the natural energy generated by the ocean to everyone who was enjoying it.

She smelled things she had never been aware of before—the smell of the water; the smell of the heat generated from the sun; the tanning preparations that were used and the aromas from food.

She listened to the tranquil sound of the ocean rolling onto the beach; the sea gulls talking to each other; and the music people were listening to. And laughter—there was so much laughter.

She tasted the salt from the water as it splashed her face and did not even mind the sand that accompanied it. She savored the feel of a cold beverage quenching her thirst on a hot day.

She felt things she had never felt before—the way the sand molded to her body when she laid on it, not even caring if it got in her swim suit; the swirling of the sand beneath her feet as the ocean would erase her footsteps; the power of the water from the ocean; the warmth of the sun; the breeze that blew through her hair. She also felt the presence of love as she looked into Vern's eyes.

"I feel like I have come back from the dead, Vern. People take so many things for granted. I know I did before. Being away from this for so long was hard, but if the reason was to reach this stage of awareness, it was worth it."

As Patty proceeded to climb up the mountain to her castle, she was not sliding back. She would not let herself. Then one day I could not believe my ears when I heard Vern call Patty, PRINCESS. She looked at him in complete amazement as she related Dr. Lagoutaris' interpretation of the mountain, the climb, and the castle. She would be the princess of her castle; she had never thought of that before until Vern called her that. She was feeling a strong sense of accomplishment because she was reaching her castle. She was almost there. Princess was not the only name Vern called Patty. He called her ISIS, too. I have heard that these terms of endearments that humans call each other are called pet names. What I did not understand was that, as smart as Vern is, he did not know I was the pet and Patty was the human. Sometimes I do not understand humans.

The three of us did almost everything together. My list of human friends was growing. I got to meet Vern and Bill's mother, Dorothy. I also met Carol, Bill's girlfriend, and she would bring me treats when she would come over to see us. She talked about how special her doggie, Panda, was and I liked her from the moment I met her. She really had a lot of feelings for animals. I could tell from what she said about Panda. Panda was a beagle and their job is usually hunting. Panda did not have to work though; her job turned out to be Carol's friend.

Among my new animal friends was Mattie, Flo and Leonard's dog. Linny and Gary had also adopted Kelsey. I liked them both, but I did let them know that I had seniority. There were many picnics, parties, and get-togethers. One thing I can say about humans is that they use any reason to have a get-together. This sure beats Patty and me being home alone.

One day in March 1990, Vern was all excited because he said he had a surprise for Patty. I was looking for a box or a bag because Vern was always surprising Patty with presents. I didn't see anything. What could the surprise be? He said, "What would you think about spending the whole summer in Ocean City, Maryland?" Patty and I listened as Vern told us about the summer job he was offered. Then he looked at me and said, "Guess what, Scruffy, you are going too."

All I have to hear are the words CAR, GO, or GOING and my ears stand straight up at attention and my tail starts wagging. I always knew Vern loved me because he would give me baths and take me for walks. He would give me manicures, buy me presents, and get me Dairy Queen cones. I also had to humor him when he would play war games with me by throwing pillows he called missiles, and I had to move very fast to miss getting bombed. Then there was the time he arranged my curl on top of my head into a Mohawk and colored it with a fluorescent green magic marker. He had taken me on a lot of car rides, but never on vacation with Patty and him. I was so excited to learn I was going, and as I looked at Patty, I knew I was ready.

Patty, on the other paw, looked like she was deep in thought. During the last two years she had been doing so much. Driving back and forth to Erie was a major accomplishment alone. Vern and she had taken vacations to Cleveland; Virginia Beach; Norfolk; Buffalo; Williamsburg, Virginia; Niagara Falls; and Toronto. They had attended plays, concerts, football games, hockey games, and many parties, and all had gone well. These times were not panic free, but by concentrating on her breathing, going through the alphabet thinking of different words and snapping her rubber band to keep herself in the present, she would get through the panic attack without having to retreat. She always knew in her mind that she would be home again in her safe place. Being nine hours away from her safe place for the whole summer was another story. It is very hard for anyone who has not suffered panic disorder with agoraphobia to understand the continuous process of having to work on your positive self-talk.

Patty had continued to see Dr. Lagoutaris, but she did not have to go as often since her medication had been regulated. It was amazing that with the behavior modification and new positive thinking, her medication was dramatically reduced. Two of the three medications were even discontinued. Patty had also been seeing Dr. Mary DeAngelis, a therapist, for almost a year.

Living life had changed so much in the past ten years. Patty had taken a break from living life, but time stands still for no one and even the new products that had hit the market had shown her this. Televisions were now accompanied with VCRs, and video stores were a booming new business. Cameras were not the only way to keep memories alive since the camcorder had been introduced. Audiotapes, that were formerly 8-tracks, were now smaller and called cassettes. Computers were fast becoming a household necessity, and not only did humans give you their telephone number but also their fax numbers.

There were other discoveries that also had an impact on how humans had to make changes in their lives during the last decade. The medical authorities had alerted humans about herpes and humans were dying from a disease called Aids. Smoking was no longer fashionable, but an addiction and habit. Violence was at an all time high with drive-by shootings and car jacking being everyday news stories.

Patty told Dr. DeAngelis that she had been changing her self-talk and practicing what she had learned from cognitive behavioral therapy.

Dr. DeAngelis explained rational fear was different than panic disorder fear, which becomes irrational.

Patty had also been concerned that, for a while, she had been labeled manic.

Dr. DeAngelis suggested that, possibly, she was not a true manic but had a single episode that reflected manic features. Patty had told Dr. DeAngelis that this had been a valuable lesson for her. Any medication—whether prescribed or over the counter—should have very detailed information obtained from the pharmacist. Patty found that they were more than happy to help you. Patty found so many humans who cared and wanted to help, but the secret to recovering was her responsibility to help herself. She wanted to know everything she could about panic disorder and any new ideas that could limit them. Dr. DeAngelis told Patty to picture a big red STOP sign if she started her WHAT-IF thinking. Life is a precious gift and our Creator wants everyone to be happy. I think that is why certain humans are given certain talents to help other humans.

Vern, knowing Patty as well as me, said, "Patty, I could always bring you home. I know how much you love the ocean and Scruffy will be with us. We will take a weekend to go down so you can familiarize yourself with the area so you will have a mental picture, and you can always call Dr. DeAngelis or Dr. Lagoutaris if need be."

I have said it before, but I must say it again, that Vern was so smart because that was all it took. A big smile lit up Patty's face and she said, "I can't believe it, the whole summer at the ocean."

Dr. Baker and his veterinarian assistants could not believe Support Dog Scruffy, who had been in the house too until Patty started going out, was going to Ocean City for the summer. Dr. Baker even said, "Scruffy, I think you should take me with you so you will have your own personal veterinarian with you."

The WHAT-IF thinking that Patty was trying to control sometimes has its advantages. She wanted to make sure I was in good health for the trip and she wanted to get a copy of my medical records. This was a good idea, I thought, in case I had to see a veterinarian in Ocean City so they would not be giving me any shots I already had.

The day finally came and after we successfully made room in the car for everything we wanted to take, I went on the longest ride I had ever taken. I was having so much fun and I did not sleep the entire way. I was too busy looking out the window. I do not know how Patty stayed in the house for all those years. There is so much out here to see. Vern was fun to travel with because he would always point out when we were nearing some horses, cows, or other animals. I would just let him think he saw them first.

We pulled up in a driveway and Vern turned off the car

saying we were there. I could see a white building that had a porch in front and a garage attached to the side. There were three pine trees in the front yard and the grass had sand mixed through it. Along the other side of the building were steps that led upstairs to another porch that extended the length of the squared structure. When I started up the steps Vern said, "Scruffy, we are down here." I thought that was good because if I wanted to go outside it would be closer.

Once inside our summer home, I noticed all the walls were knotty pine. It reminded Patty and Vern of a cabin, but with all the modern conveniences. It was cozy and perfect for us. I could tell Patty felt comfortable immediately.

After a good night's sleep, the first thing Patty and Vern did was move the table away from the front window and put the couch there so I could get a good view. They sure are good to me. Then Vern took Patty to acquaint her with the area. He showed her the drug store, laundromat, grocery store, post office, video store, and dry cleaners—all the places humans need to go. They also took a walk to the ocean, which was only a block away from our summer home.

Everything was within walking distance. Walking was still hard for Patty because she felt the farther she walked the longer it would take her to get back home if it were necessary. However, this location was so centrally located that she felt safe wherever she walked. She had taken her weights to exercise and using her visualization, positive thinking, and behavior modification. Patty continually worked on what had become her new way of life, but I noticed she was also drawing on the strength she found in Vern and the ocean. She started walking the boardwalk every morning. Vern would run every other day, and on those days they had a designated bench on the boardwalk where they would meet, have coffee and just watch the humans passing by. Patty told Vern that even seeing the ocean every day, she was still in awe of its wonder.

There were rules about what months dogs could be on the boardwalk and beaches, but that did not stop Vern. He checked to see what beaches allowed dogs. He was becoming dog's best friend, or at least one of mine. We decided to go to Assateague Island which had many beaches. Assateague was also famous because of the wild horses that lived there and roamed the island. So, not only was I going to the beach to swim, but also I was seeing horses walk in front of the car and along the sides of the road. I like horses, after all *Mr. Ed* is one of my favorite television shows. I wonder if he is here!

Vern took a while to find just the right spot before we laid a blanket down, put a big umbrella up and arranged the cooler and other treats humans take to the beach. Patty and Vern remembered everything including my water dish. Vern picked me up as we headed toward the ocean. While carrying me he is saying, "Scruffy, look at this big bathtub."

Well, I do not know what bathtub he has taken baths in but I had never seen one like this! It went as far as my eyes could see right to the sky and there were rolling waves of water that made very big splashes. He carried me as he started walking in the water. Patty stood and watched from the sandy area that met the water. I knew she was concerned whether or not I knew how to swim. The water was up to Vern's waist when he turned and let me go. It was lots of fun swimming through the waves back to Patty. I barked and jumped up and down to let them know I wanted to do it again. I knew I looked a sight and that my curl on my head had seen better days, but I didn't care, this was fun. So Vern did it again and again. Then it was time to rest.

I drew a crowd of beach humans when I started digging for crabs in the sand. I don't mind telling you I made that sand fly high to get what I wanted. I can now understand why the ocean was so special to Patty. She was so happy and calm as she looked mesmerized at the water coming up to the beach. She was a different human than the person I met six years ago.

I had done so many things with Vern. He had taken me to the mountain where he hunts deer. He even let me help him look for tracks. Oh, he knew I was a Support Dog but some humans have two jobs. Maybe I could be a hunting dog, too. Vern had also taken me and Patty boating. There all the human boaters laughed when I dove off the dock to chase some ducks. It happened so fast that when I realized what I had done, I swam back to the dock. My buddy Vern was there to rescue me and lift me back up on the dock. Everything that has been created is so unique, but the Creator went out of His way with this ocean. My time at the ocean was really special to me. The peacefulness made me forget that sometimes it could be a dog-eat-dog world out there. I am glad Vern was sent into our lives.

There were many new humans I met that summer. Another good reason Patty had to get on with her life and get out of her house, not only because of what she had been missing but who she had been missing. There are humans you meet that touch your life for a brief encounter. Then there are humans you meet that you know will be a part of your life forever. This is how I felt when I met Laura, Vern's daughter, who came to stay with us. Humans sometimes call the kind of eyes Laura has, cat eyes. I knew immediately when I met Laura that she loved dogs because I heard her say she dog-sat for doggies that were not as fortunate as me to go on vacation with their masters. I also knew Patty really liked her. When Vern was working, Laura and Patty spent their time together. I do not know how humans can talk so much but Laura and Patty talked about everything. There was lots of laughing, too, which I always wished I could do because it sure makes humans happy when they do it. Laura did not eat red meat, and that summer she taught Patty so many different ways chicken could be served. Patty would laugh as she would tell Vern, "Well, I learned my 1,000th way to order chicken today."

On the day Laura was to fly back to Florida I noticed tears in her beautiful eyes. I wanted to say, "Laura, be happy, everything will be fine and don't worry, you will see us again. You are one of our favorite friends."

Vern and Patty took Laura to the airport, and as Patty waved good-bye the airplane took off. Patty wondered, "Will I ever try and fly again? I do not know how I will, because I still feel very anxious just being here in the airport. Oh, well, there are many people who choose another way to travel rather than fly. I can live a full life without flying again."

Since Ocean City is a resort town, most humans came for a week or two and then went home. Vern's cousin and her family came from New Jersey and stayed right on top of us. We would all sit on the porches and the humans would talk. I, on the other paw, would be checking out what was going on in the neighborhood. There were lots of cookouts and I heard someone say they were having hot dogs and hamburgers. I never could understand why humans call their food hot dogs. We don't call our food "hot humans."

There were a lot of college students working in Ocean City for the summer. Their pets were not as lucky as I was because they had to stay home. It was not long before the college humans that were staying by us, adopted me. Since we spent much of our time outside, they would stop and talk to me. I knew I was the popular one between the three of us because even if Vern and Patty were inside, the college humans would sit and play with me. I heard one tell Patty, "We have all adopted Scruffy as the neighborhood pet." Patty would be walking back from the post office and she would be asked, "When is Scruffy coming outside?" There were times we were in the house watching videos and there would be a knock on the door. Vern would answer the door and someone would ask, "Can Scruffy come out and play?" Vern would say, "Scruffy is resting right now, maybe a little later." I hope he isn't feeling insecure about my love for him. After all, we have a common interest in Patty. I better go give him some extra kisses. The manager where we stayed had a granddaughter who would play with me. She would ask, "Where did you get that curl on top of your head, Scruffy?" Then there was Peck, an elderly gentle human who lived across from us. He came over a couple of times a day to see me. He was always bringing me treats and I am not talking regular treats. He would bring crab cakes. I would get so excited when I saw him coming. I loved him and I knew he loved me. One day, Patty and Vern were cooking hamburgers on the grill. Peck came over and I knew he had something that was wrapped up in his hands. He said, "Does Scruffy like lobster?" Patty and Vern looked at each other, then down at their hamburgers and started laughing. As I feasted on lobster Vern said, "Scruffy, you better not even look at me while I am eating my hamburger." I know humans say the dog days of August, but for me it was a dog's summer here.

I also had one dog friend who lived in Ocean City all year-long, by the name of Skipper. He was one good-looking Cocker Spaniel and I knew he liked me too. His master would walk him every day and you could bet I knew when he was a block away. I usually was outside, but if I wasn't I made it known I had to go outside so I could see him. This must be puppy love because I have never been so taken by another dog.

We had so much fun that we spent the next summer there, too. It is funny how, even if you have to leave someplace, the memories are with you forever. Patty had grown so much stronger. It was a miracle. Vern and I were so proud of her. I had been with her so I knew what she went through. However, if you had just met this tanned blonde, blue-eyed human who had lost all that weight you wouldn't think she ever had a care in the world. She looked radiant. She grew with every step she took during recovery, but there was something magical about the ocean that made such a difference in her. Vern was a big help to my mission and I thank him, and my Creator for sending Vern into our lives.

CHAPTER 10

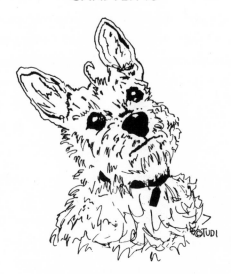

There have been many times during the almost nine years that we have been together that Patty would ask me, "Scruffy, where did you come from? You are an angel, aren't you? You do know how much you have helped me?"

I would just look at her and remind myself that some things are best left unsaid.

Thank goodness therapy is so much more accepted now than it was before. Humans never think twice about a diabetic having to take medication. The way I look at it, if a human had a broken leg no one would think anything about that human getting medical attention. If you didn't get medical attention everyone would think you were irresponsible because the break wouldn't heal right and you might have a limp, among other complications. Mental illness, not given proper medical attention, could cause one to limp through life. I know one of the most important lessons Patty learned was that to be a complete human, you had to work on your MIND, BODY and SPIRIT. When there is a problem with one area, you can be sure there will be subsequent problems in the other areas.

Dr. DeAngelis became a positive force in Patty's life by helping Patty continue her climb to her castle. Patty thought agoraphobia was the fear of wide-open spaces like shopping malls or auditoriums. After all it was defined as the fear of the market place. "Why then," Patty asked, "the panic attack in the airplane almost sixteen years ago? Do you think I have claustrophobia, too? The area in the airplane was not that wide open."

Dr. DeAngelis explained that one of the symptoms of agoraphobia was the fear of losing control whether the area was large or small.

Patty remembered back to one of her more recent panic attacks, which became full blown on her one to ten scale.

Her sister Tudi was getting married. Patty was honored that she was asked to be the maid of honor at the wedding. Humans, I have noticed, get very emotional when there is an approaching wedding but Patty was handling the situation well.

She was familiar with the church where the wedding would take place. She even made visits to the church to reestablish where the exits were. Her self-talk was telling her the ceremony would last thirty minutes, which was not that long. Linny, her other sister, was matron of honor, so between her and Tudi she would feel safe. The upcoming walk down the aisle was not making her happy. She said she would rather be in position when the wedding started; the aisle was not long— she could do it.

At the rehearsal the night before, Patty found out she would be on the altar with the bride and groom and the best man for the entire ceremony. Linny would be in the first pew of the church with the flower girl. She immediately started WHAT-IF I get sick; WHAT-IF I have to leave; WHAT-IF I faint; WHAT-IF I cannot remember what I have to do; and the WHAT-IFs just continued to mount. I heard she was thinking of dropping out of the wedding and not even attending. I know she was in a lot of turmoil because she really loved Tudi.

Leonard told Patty that her position on the altar was better than sitting in the first pew. He said if she had to leave there was an exit to the left, and that Linny would notice and be able to step into Patty's place. Something so simple, yet it was all she needed. That night, being her Support Dog, I stayed close to her and let her draw strength from me by cuddling. The wedding was beautiful and you know what? Patty did not have to leave at all. I still bark at the thought of those

WHAT-IFs. They are the worst things a human can think or say. However, with every setback, Patty was more determined and would learn something from each trial she experienced. She concentrated harder on abolishing the WHAT-IFs from her vocabulary.

Dr. Fridley started the process of fulfilling Patty's dream of having a perfect smile. The process would take almost six months, and he knew she was ready. Together with his colleague, Dr. Generalovich, there were sometimes eight-hour appointments. I knew she was doing better with her self-talk now. Gosh, I know humans who do not suffer from panic disorder who would have a panic attack sitting in a dentist chair that long. When the work had been completed Patty smiled more than ever. Her new smile represented the new way she looked at life, not the telltale signs of medications she had been prescribed in unhappy times. This was done at a good time because Patty was happy with herself and how well she had been doing. Her blue eyes were not the only things that sparkled now. Her white teeth sparkled, too.

Yes, I sure had seen a change in Patty from when I had first met her. She would no longer just sit in her house and wait for things to change. Instead, she worked on changing the things she wanted to change. When Ross Perot said he would run for president if his name were put on the ballot in all fifty states, Patty searched for a local group who supported him.

She found that group, attended the meeting for Mercer County, and that was the first time she did not seek out someone to go with her. She came back all excited and said, "Scruffy, I am the Petition Coordinator for Mercer County. I have to take one day at a time but I can do it. Do you believe I am now an Agoraphobic Activist?" She said, "While I was in the house the United States went into a four trillion dollar deficit. I feel I must try and help this country by doing my part."

One of her highest moments was when she was able to see Mr. Perot in Pittsburgh. She would not let the WHAT-IFs ruin this opportunity. She just went. When Patty voted, the tears rolled down her cheeks because she knew she had played a part in getting his name on the ballot.

Yes, I had a good assignment. Sure it was rough at first, but the rewards were big ones. I had been treated like a pedigree and even more than treats, I had been given so much love. It was well worth it even if before every Christmas I was dressed up like Santa, a reindeer, an angel, or some other Christmas theme for our annual Christmas card. Humans come up with some pretty strange ideas sometimes.

Patty was living her dreams now. The activities she had visualized were becoming a reality now. She had been to the ocean, seen *Mickey Mouse on Ice*, had attended Diana Ross, Johnny Mathis and Neil Diamond concerts. She had seen a performance of the play *Cats* and she was traveling at least by car.

She still had panic attacks and was a recovering agoraphobic, but she was in control. Exercise, proper rest, spacing activities, avoiding caffeine and diet products with aspartame were all helpful in controlling anxiety and panic. When she did have a panic attack she would let it happen, concentrate on her breathing and divert her thinking so it wouldn't last any longer than necessary.

She now looked at the panic and listened to what it was trying to tell her. Slow down—get some rest. Stop eating those chocolate candy bars. Too much stress—go exercise.

This was not just something you learned and did not put into practice. It was the new way Patty lived life. I thought it was a doggoned good way to live, too. It was time to ask the Creator to take her further.

Patty and her friend, Carol, had made reservations to attend a Ladies' Day Out where you picked two lectures out of a variety of subjects. They were told when they made their reservations to choose a third topic as a substitute in case their first two selections were filled. Patty picked Decorating with Color and Are You Listening? Her third choice was Dream Vacations. Okay, so she was visualizing. Sure she had traveled by car, but this lecture was to be given by a travel agent and was about air trips and cruises.

I knew I needed all the help I could get for this last final hurdle up her mountain to her castle, to get her in an airplane again. So once again I went to my Creator. I know I do that a lot, but we are told to "ask and we shall receive." I always give thanks for my answers, too. I wonder if I say thanks enough.

Dr. DeAngelis explained to Patty that getting on an airplane again was what she still feared the most because that was where her first full-blown panic attack had occurred.

Things were taken out of my paws that day in April when both Carol and Patty attended the lecture on Dream Vacations because Decorating with Color was filled. Patty listened about all the places that awaited her by airplane and cruise ships. The thirty-minute ride home from their Ladies' Day Out, Carol and Patty reflected back on their day.

They laughed at the fun they had and then Patty got serious. Patty told Carol she would love to take a cruise, being surrounded by the ocean.

A cruise would mean flying to get you to the ship. Carol said, "Patty, you can do anything you want. You are much stronger than you even know."

Patty told Carol she had been practicing to travel by airplane again. She had driven to the airport and sat in the airport parking lot. On a later excursion she proved she could go inside the airport and have a cup of coffee. She had gone again and again each time staying a little longer. Laughing, she told Carol, "There were times I was concerned because I thought the airport personnel would think I was casing the place, after all I never went anywhere nor was I picking anyone up or dropping anyone off. Then I started taking family and friends to the airport for trips they were taking so I did not look so suspicious. What will it take to get me to fly again? Someday I will call that travel agent we listened to today."

The very next day in the mail Patty received an invitation to Laura's college graduation in Florida. She had known it was coming. Laura had been talking about graduation for a year now. She had been asking Patty to come since November to share this day with her. Ever since Ocean City three years before when Patty and Laura first met, their friendship continued to grow. I knew Laura was very special to Patty because I had heard her say to Laura, "If you ever need me just call, I will always be here for you."

Patty looked at the invitation, then at me and said, "Scruffy, I have always told Laura I would be here for her. Well, she does not want me here—she wants me in Florida at her graduation."

She went to the telephone and dialed and I heard her say, "Vern, I just received my invitation for Laura's graduation. I want to go. What are your flight arrangements?"

I could not believe my ears. Patty was facing her final fear! I got real close to her because I knew my buddy, Vern, had to be as surprised as me and I wanted to hear what he said, which was, "You are ready, aren't you?" I could not believe he was not even surprised. He couldn't know Patty better than me. Could he? No, he was just in shock.

Since he was at school, he called Patty back with the information. He was flying from Erie to Pittsburgh then to Florida. Patty said she would rather catch the flight in Pittsburgh so that way she could not get off before they landed in Orlando. Since Vern had scheduled his flight a week before and he would already be on the airplane first, he said he would make sure their seats were together. Vern said, "Call the travel agency to make sure you can get on this flight." He also told Patty to concentrate on how happy Laura would be and not to overdo it before the trip, which was two weeks and one day away. He said he would be in to celebrate Patty's birthday on Sunday and they would call and tell Laura together.

She called the travel agent she had spoken with the day before and made the arrangements. When she got off the telephone she said, "Scruffy, just yesterday I said someday I would make this call. I thought of the old saying, 'Don't put off tomorrow what you could do today'." She went on to say, "I wondered what it would take to get me to fly again. It was Laura."

Reality set in. WHAT HAD SHE DONE? "Now calm down. You are in control," she told herself. "You can cancel at any time and Vern would understand." She knew, however, that once they told Laura she would be so excited she couldn't back out.

Vern came to take everyone out to dinner to celebrate Patty's birthday. He knew she liked birthdays as much as Christmas—well almost.

When she opened her present from Vern he said that the other part of her present was a trip to see Mickey Mouse in Disney World while they were in Florida. It was as if he was giving her an added incentive.

When I heard that, I knew there was no stopping her. Patty would not only be seeing Laura but Mickey Mouse.

The next two weeks were busy ones, not only physically getting ready for the trip but also preparing mentally and spiritually.

THE FIRST THING was positive affirmations (she repeated these several times a day):

— I am totally relaxed and in control

— I am going to the airport in complete control of my thoughts and emotions

— I AM CALM! I AM RELAXED!

— I board the plane with ease—I am opening up all opportunities to myself...I am calm!

— I want to fly and see the beauty of the sky...the clouds...

— I AM SAFE...I AM RELAXED...I AM CALM ... I AM READY...

— I AM HAPPY![1]

Patty counteracted every WHAT-IF that crossed her mind. She went to talk to the pharmacist knowing that even over-the-counter medications could cause excitability or depression. She wanted to be prepared just in case the flight caused any congestion or motion sickness. Patty never chewed gum, but she bought some. A *Word Search Puzzle* book was purchased to divert her thinking. Patty packed all these items in a carry-on that she called her SELF-HELP TO GET ME THROUGH THE FLIGHT BAG. She went to Dr. DeAngelis for a couple of sessions, where the therapist talked about what to expect on the flight.

Dr. DeAngelis told her to take her headset on the trip and gave her a tape called *Relax—Let Go—Relax*.[2] They practiced breathing. Slowly breathing in calmness through her nose, slowly blowing out anxiety through her mouth. She also told Patty to refresh Vern's memory on the breathing exercise in case she became anxious and forgot to concentrate on her breathing, he could remind her.

The flight was leaving at 8:15 a.m., May 8th. Tudi picked us up at 6:00 a.m. I was going on a little vacation myself because I was going to stay with her. Believe me, I was ready for a vacation after a hectic two weeks of seeing Patty getting ready.

Vern had called almost everyday to make sure Patty was not overdoing. There were days I wished I could have taken the phone and talked to him. After all, I do need my beauty sleep.

Tudi was teasing Patty on the way to the airport that if she did not want to go she would take her place and go with Vern to Florida. She laughed saying Vern probably would not like her company as well, but that would be his problem.

Patty told Tudi that she felt surprisingly calm. She also went on to say, "When I had that big panic attack sixteen years ago I had no idea what it was, now I know, and I <u>know</u> how to deal with it. I have gotten ready PHYSICALLY, MENTALLY and SPIRITUALLY.

I have said three novenas, and an order of nuns in Erie who dedicate their lives to praying for others, are all praying for U.S. Air Flight 201. I am even carrying a prayer that says, "Whoever reads this prayer or hears it or carries it will never die a sudden death, nor be drowned, nor will poison take effect on them. They will not fall into the hands of the enemy nor be burned in any fire, nor will they be defeated in battle." [3]

Tudi laughed saying, "Vern has no idea how safe he is flying with you, Patty."

We approached the airport and Tudi pulled over to let Patty out. Patty kissed me good-bye and said, "Well, Scruffy, I am going to Florida. I am ready. Be good for Tudi. I love you."

I knew she was ready. She had a look of confidence on her face. "I love you, too, Patty," I barked. "You have fun. Tell Laura and Vern I said hello. Don't worry, I will be good."

Tudi told me, as she parked the car, that they were going to check Patty's luggage — all except her carry-on of SELF-HELP TO GET ME THROUGH THE FLIGHT BAG. They would then go to the reservation desk to check in for her flight. Well, this should be fairly easy because Patty had visualized this many times. Tudi parked the car and said she would be back soon and would tell me everything that happened.

"Don't worry, Scruffy," she said, "she will get on the airplane and she will be fine."

I thought she would get on the plane. I just wanted her flight to be panic free. She had her rubber band on her wrist to keep her mind focused in the present. A thought crossed my mind, wouldn't it be something if someone from the crew on her last "fright flight" was on this trip? Oh, I got up so early today I should lie down for a while. No way, I have to look out the window. There sure is a lot of activity here. I see Tudi coming back to the car. It is just Tudi! PATTY DID IT! I started barking. I was so excited.

Tudi spoke as she got into the car, "Scruffy, you would have been proud. Patty was a little anxious when Flight 201 landed from Erie. Before she boarded the plane we were going through the alphabet to divert her thinking when we looked up and there was Vern. He had received permission to get off the plane so he could board with Patty."

Why didn't that surprise me? That Vern is one great male human and I know how protective he is of Patty.

Tudi said the last thing they did before they boarded the airplane was made sure Vern remembered the breathing exercise.

"Vern breathed with Patty and started laughing saying, 'Patty, you are not having a baby. You are going to Florida to see Laura and Mickey Mouse.' We said our good-byes, and Patty boarded like she had been doing this every day. You would have been proud."

As we watched the airplane take off, I knew she would be fine. I knew Vern would make sure of that. I knew she would not need a thing from her SELF-HELP TO GET ME THROUGH THE FLIGHT BAG. I knew she would cry because she would be happy that her last obstacle had been defeated. I WOULD BET dog treats, that as Flight 201 soared to its cruising altitude, she would remember their song. She would say to Vern, "I can fly higher than an eagle, for you are the wind beneath my wings; thank you, thank you, thank God for you are the wind beneath my wings." [4]

When Patty came home, she told me she loved flying again. The flight attendant had given her a puppet airplane that had playing cards inside and more than that, a set of wings for flying again.

She told me all about Laura and her graduation which was

held in a huge auditorium that Patty would not have been able to attend a few years ago.

She told me about the party given after Laura graduated and how she got to meet the humans that Laura had talked about.

Patty told me that not only did she see Mickey Mouse, he had kissed her. Then afterward, how Vern and she had to sit down because she was crying so hard over her happiness.

How they laughed when she said that everyone probably thought they were fighting because she was crying so hard!

They had gone on all the rides, which would have been impossible with her old WHAT-IF way of thinking.

Patty went on to say that the phrase IF YOU DREAM IT-IT CAN HAPPEN was at the exit of one of the rides.

A miracle, I thought, because like anyone who is close to Patty, I knew, this was her big dream come true.

She did have panic attacks while she was there, but was in control of them. She knew it was because of the excitement and the lack of sleep. Patty told me how Vern, on the flight home, said that this trip was like a graduation for her too. He knew she was different than when they first met. She had developed determination and strength beyond belief. Patty had fought hard to win her battle and she had won. I knew she was determined to get to the top of that mountain to her castle and she did. The climb was not always easy. I know because I scampered right beside her. Patty had faced her fears to free herself. I looked at her and saw so much courage.

She works at being the best she can be so she is free to live again. I love her and I know she loves me so very much, and I thank my Creator every day for my pawsitive mission.

My duties as Support Dog continue since recovery is an ongoing process, so this is not the end. No, there will be no retirement for me because I will stand by my human as she continues her new beginning. When I think of how far Patty has come, I just want to bark to the world, "We were in—but now we are OUT!"

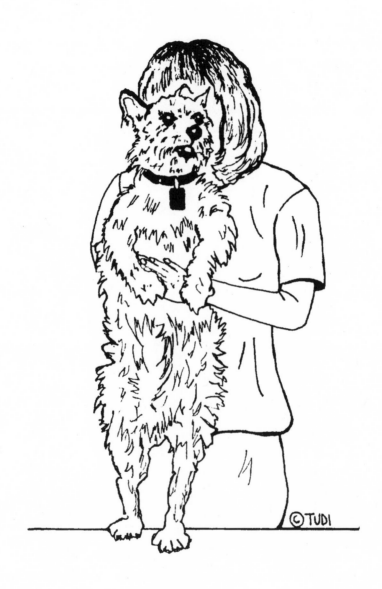

APPENDICES

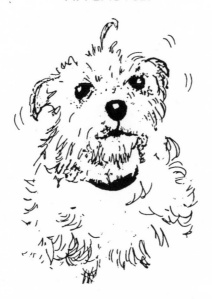

APPENDIX - A

Scruffy's Pawsitive Tips

1. Make an appointment for a complete physical to rule out any physical causes for panicky feelings.

2. Find a psychologist who is knowledgeable about Panic Disorder. One who uses relaxation and Behavior Modification techniques is recommended.

3. To locate the most qualified professionals:

   a. Contact your family doctor. He will recommend a psychologist who is knowledgeable about Panic Disorder. If medication is needed, the psychologist will recommend a psychiatrist.

   b. Your clergyman may be helpful in suggesting a professional.

   c. Contact help-information centers at your local hospitals.

   d. A person who has received therapy is a good source of information.

4. ALWAYS, ALWAYS REMEMBER—you have the right to change your therapist or get a second, third or fourth opinion.

5. Continue learning everything you can about Panic Disorder by reading, attending lectures and workshops.

6. Every time you say WHAT-IF, tell yourself to STOP.

7. Replace old self-talk with positive talk by reading positive thinking books and listening to positive audiotapes. Learn to visualize yourself being panic free.

8. Face your fears gradually, give yourself permission to retreat WITH-OUT being critical of yourself and PRAISE yourself for each accomplishment.

9. To relax:

    a. Learn to relax by breathing in calmness SLOWLY through your nose—exhaling anxiety so softly that a candle flame will not even flicker.

    b. Wear a rubber band on your wrist and snap it if you start the WHAT-IFs in order to remain focused on the present.

    c. Go through the alphabet to divert thinking by reciting three-letter words-for example, ate, bet, cat, dog, —then four-letter words, etc.

10. Make exercising a part of your life, make sure you get your proper rest and learn to space your activities.

11. Avoid caffeine and diet products with aspartame. Know that your pharmacists are very knowledgeable and helpful. Consult them before taking any over-the-counter medications, and ask any questions you have about your prescriptions.

12. Visit your doctor's office to make appointments so you can have a visual picture and explain your Panic Disorder to the staff.

13. Ask for the first appointment of the day so you do not have to wait long so you do not have to think about the appointment all day.

14. Take someone with you for support to your appointments.

15. Learn to laugh, laugh a lot. Humor is sometimes the best medicine.

16. And above all, don't forget that a pet can be a real source of support and strength. People who have pets are healthier, live longer, and have fewer stress-related illnesses.

APPENDIX - B

Phobias Listed by Objects of Fear [1]

Afraid, being—Phobophobia
Age, old—Gerontophobia
Airplanes—Pterygephobia
Alcohol—Dipsophobia; Methyphobia
Alone, being—Autophobia; Eremiophobia; Monophobia
Animal fur—Doraphobia
Animals—Zoophobia
Bacilli—Bacillophobia
      (see Microbiophobia, fear of germs)
Bacteria—Bacteriophobia
      (see Microbiophobia, fear of germs)
Baldness, bald people—Peladophobia
Beaten, being—Mastigophobia; Rhabdophobia
Bed, staying in—Klinocophobia
Bees—Apiphobia; Melissophobia
Bicycles—Cyclophobia
Birds-Ornithophobia
Births, giving—Lochiophobia; Maieusophobia; Tocophobia
Birth defects—Teratophobia
      (see Dysmorphophobia, fear of deformed people)
Black—Melanophobia
Blindness, going blind, blind people—Typhlophobia
Blood, sight of—Hematophobia; Hemophobia
Blue—Caerulephobia
Blushing-Eurethrophobia
Body odors—Bromidrosi-; Bromidrosiphobia
Books—Bibliophobia
Bound, being—Merintophobia
Brain diseases—Meningitophobia
Breezes—Aerophobia

Bridges, crossing-Gephyrophobia
Bullets—Ballistophobia
Bulls—Boustrophobia
Burglars—Clepto-; Kleptophobia; Harpaxophobia
Buried alive, being—Taphephobia
Cadavers—Necrophobia
               (see Thanatophobia, fear of death)
Cancer—Cancerophobia
Cats—Ailurophobia; Galeophobia; Gatophobia
Cattle-Boustrophobia
Change—Metathesiophobia; Caeno-; Caino-;
           Cainto-;Kaino-; Kainotophobia; Neophobia
Childbirth—Lochiophobia; Maieusophobia; Tocophobia
Children—Pedophobia
Chins—Geniophobia
Choking—Pnigero-; Pnigophobia
Cholera—Cholerophobia
Church—Hagiophobia; Hierophobia
Cities—Cosmophobia; Polisophobia
Clawed, being—Amychophobia
Cliffs—Cremnophobia
Clocks—Chronophobia
Close relationships—Philophobia
Coitus—Coitophobia; Erotophobia
Cold—Cheimophobia; Cryophobia
Colors, various—Chromato-; Chromophobia
          Black—Melanophobia
          Blue—Caerulephobia
          Gold—Chrysophobia
          Green—Chlorephobia
          Purple—Porphyrophobia
          Red—Erythrophobia
          Yellow—Xanthophobia
          White—Leucophobia
Comets—Cometophobia
Confined spaces—Claustrophobia

Contact, physical—Aphe-; Haphe-; Haptephobia
Contamination—Molysmophobia; Mysophobia; Rhypophobia
Corpses—Necrophobia
      (see Thanatophobia, fear of death)
Courts—Dikephobia
Cows—Boustrophobia
Crossing bridges—Gephyrophobia
Crossing streets—Agyiophobia; Dromophobia
Crowds—Demophobia; Koinoniphobia; Ochlophobia
Cut, being—Amychophobia
Dampness—Hygrophobia
Dancing—Chorophobia
Darkness—Achluophobia; Nocti-; Nyctophobia; Scotophobia
Dawn—Cosophobia
Daylight—Phengophobia
Dead bodies—Necrophobia
Death—Thanatophobia
Deep water—Batho-; Bathyphobia
Defecation—Coprophobia
Defects, birth—Teratophobia
Deformities—Teratophobia
Deformed people—Dysmorphophobia
Demons—Daemono-; Demonophobia
Dentists—Odontiatrophobia
Desolate places—Kenophobia; Topophobia
Destructive actions—Ergasiophobia
Devils—Daemono-; Demonophobia
Diabetes—Diabetophobia
Dirges—Threnatophobia
Dirt—Molysmophobia; Mysophobia; Rhypo-; Rupophobia
Diseases, various—Nosophobia; Pathophobia
      Alcoholism—Dipsophobia
      Brain diseases—Meningitophobia
      Cancer—Cancerophobia
      Cholera—Cholerophobia
      Diabetes—Diabetophobia

Diseases, various (continued)—
>
> Hair diseases—Trichopathophobia
> Heart diseases—Cardiophobia
> Insanity—Dementophobia; Lyssophobia
> Intestinal diseases—Enterophobia
> Meningitis—Meningitophobia
> Rabies—Hydrophobophobia; Lyssophobia
> Skin diseases—Dermatopatho;Dermatosiophobia
> Tapeworm infestation—Taeniophobia
> Tetanus—Tetanophobia
> Trichinosis—Trichinophobia
> Tuberculosis—Phthisiophobia; Tuberculophobia
> Venereal diseases—Cypridophobia;
> > Syphilophobia;
> > Venereophobia

Dishonesty—Mythophobia

Disorder—Auchmophobia; Ataxiophobia; Conistraphobia

Dogs—Cynophobia

Dolls—Pediophobia

Doctors—Iatrophobia

Drafts—Aerophobia

Drugs—Pharmacophobia

Dust—Amathophobia; Coniophobia

Dummies, ventriloquists'—Pediophobia

Eating in public—Phagophobia
> (see Cibophobia; Sitophobia, fear of food)

Electricity—Electrophobia

Empty space—Kenophobia; Topophobia

Encirclement (by people)—Gyrephobia

Enclosed, being-Gyrephobia

Enclosed spaces—Claustrophobia

Error—Hamartophobia

Everything—Pano-; Pan-; Pantophobia

Evil spirits—Daemono-; Demonophobia; Phasmophobia

Exhaustion—Kopophobia

Expressing opinions—Doxophobia

Eyes—Ommatophobia
    (see Ophthalmophobia; Scopophobia, fear of being
    stared at)
Failure—Kakorrhaphiophobia
Fainting—Asthenophobia
Fat, getting; fat people—Lipophobia
Fatigue—Kopophobia
Fear—Phobophobia
Feathers—Pteronophobia
Feces—Coprophobia; Rhypo-; Rupophobia
Female genitalia—Eurotophobia
Females—Gynephobia
Fever—Febri-; Fibriphobia; Pyrexeophobia
Filth—Molysmophobia; Mysophobia; Rhypo-;
    Rupophobia
Fingers-Aichmophobia
Fire—Pyrophobia
Fish—Ichthyophobia
Flashing lights—Semaphophobia
Flavors, various—Geumatophobia
    Salty—Halophobia
    Sour—Acerbophobia
    Sweet—Hediso-; Hedysophobia
Flogged, being—Mastigophobia; Rhabdophobia
Floods—Antlophobia
Flowers—Anthophobia; Botanophobia
Flutes—Aulophobia
Flying—Pterygophobia
Fog—Homichlophobia
Food—Cibophobia; Sitophobia
    (see Phagophobia, fear of eating in public)
Forests—Hylophobia
    (see Dendrophobia, fear of trees)
Friendship—Philophobia
Frogs—Batrachophobia
Funerals—Threnatophobia

Fur, animal—Doraphobia
Gaiety—Chero-; Chorophobia
Gases—Aerophobia
Genitalia, female—Eurotophobia;
          Of either sex—Genitophobia
Germs—Bacillophobia; Bacteriophobia; Microbiophobia
Ghosts—Phasmophobia
Glaring lights—Photaugiophobia
Glass—Crystallophobia; Hyalophobia
God-Theophobia
Gold—Chrysophobia
Gravity—Barophobia
Green—Chlorephobia
Hair, hairy people—Chaetophobia; Villophobia; Trichophobia
Hair diseases—Trichopathophobia
          (see Peladophobia, fear of baldness)
Happiness—Chero-; Chorophobia
Hats—Mitrophobia
Heart disease—Cardiophobia
Heat—Thermophobia
Heaven—Uranophobia
Heights—Acrophobia; Hypsophobia
Hell—Hadephobia; Stygiophobia
Hereditary—Patroiophobia
Hidden meanings—Calyprophobia
High objects—Batophobia
High speeds—Tachyphobia
High winds—Anemophobia
Home, one's own—Oikophobia
Horses—Equinophobia
House, inside of—Domatophobia
Human society—Anthro-; Anthropophobia
Hurricanes—Anemophobia
Ideas—Ideophobia
Identity, sexual—Genophobia

Illness—Pathophobia; Nosophobia
    (see also list under "Diseases")
Infinity—Apeiro-; Apeurophobia
Inherited defects—Patroiophobia
Injury—Traumatophobia
Insects: General—Entomophobia; Small—
    Acarophobia
Instruments, wind—Aulophobia
Intercourse, sexual—Coitophobia; Erotophobia
Intestines—Enterophobia
Intestinal infestation-Taeniophobia
Jails—Dikephobia
Jealously—Zelophobia
Knives—Aichmophobia
Large bodies of water—Potaniophobia
Large objects—Megalophobia
Large (empty) spaces—Kenophobia
Learning, places of—Epistemophobia
Left side of body, objects on—Levophobia
Leprosy—Leprophobia
Libraries—Epistemophobia
    (see Bibliophobia, fear of books)
Lice—Pediculophobia; Phthiriophobia; Verminophobia
Lies—Mythophobia
Lightning—Astraphobia; Keraunophobia
Light—Photophobia
Lights: Flashing—Semaphophobia;
    Glaring-Photaugiophobia;
    Northern-Auroraphobia
Liquids—Hydrophobia
Lizards—Herpetophobia; Saurophobia
Locked in, being—Clithrophobia
Lockjaw—Tetanophobia
Loneliness—Eremio-; Eremophobia
Losing one's mind—Dementophobia
Love, sexual—Coitophobia; Erotophobia

Machinery—Mechanophobia
Males—Androphobia
Many things—Polyphobia
Marriage—Gamophobia
Mechanical objects—Mechanophobia
Medicines—Pharmacophobia
Memories—Mnemophobia
Meningitis—Meningitophobia
Metals—Metallophobia
Meteors—Meteorophobia
Mice—Musophobia
Microbes—Microbiophobia; Bacillophobia
Mirrors—Eisoptrophobia
      (see Crystallophobia; Hyalophobia, fear of glass)
Missiles—Ballistophobia
Mites—Acarophobia
Moisture—Hygrophobia
Money—Chrematophobia
      (see Chrysophobia, fear of wealth)
Moon—Selenophobia
Movement (usually rapid)—Kinesophobia
Moving (relocating)—Tropophobia
Music—Melophobia
Mushrooms—Mycophobia
Mystery—Calyprophobia
Names, certain—Onomatophobia
Narrow places—Stenophobia
Needles—Belonephobia
Nets, netting—Linonophobia
New things—Caeno-; Caino-; Cainto-; Kain
      Kainotophobia;Neophobia
Night—Achluophobia; Nocti Nyctophobia; Scotophobia
Northern lights—Auroraphobia
Nosebleeds—Epistagmophobia
Novelty—Caeno-; Caino-; Cainto-; Kaino-;
      Kainotophobia; Neophobia

Numbers, various—Numerophobia
Nudity—Gymnophobia
Obesity—Lipophobia
Objects: High—Batophobia
    Large—Megalophobia
    Pointed—Belonephobia
    Sharp—Aichmophobia
    Small—Microphobia
Obscure meanings—Calyprophobia
Oceans—Thalassophobia
Odors: Body—Bromidrosi-; Bromidrosiphobia;
Various—Olfactophobia; Osmophobia; Osphresiopshobia
Old age, old people—Gerontophobia
Oneself—Autophobia; Eremiophobia; Monophobia
Open spaces—Agoraphobia
Opinions, expressing—Doxophobia
Outer space—Astrophobia; Stratophobia
Pain—Algia-; Algophobia; Odynophobia
Parasites—Parasitophobia
People (in general)—Anthro-; Anthropophobia
Personal uncleanliness—Automysophobia
Physcial contact—Aphe-; Haphe-; Haptephobia
Physical weakness—Asthenophobia
Pins—Belonephobia
Plants—Botanophobia
Pleasure—Hedonophobia
Pointed objects—Belonephobia
Poisons—Iophobia; Toxicophob
Police—Dikephobia
Poverty—Peniaphobia
Praise, receiving—Doxophobia
Precipices—Cremnophobia
Prostitutes—Pornophobia
Public places—Agoraphobic
Punishment—Poinephobia
   (see Dikephobia, fear of justice)

Purple—Porphyrophobia
Rabies—Hydrophobophobia; Lyssophobia
Railways—Siderodromophobia
Rain—Hyetophobia; Ombrophobia
Razors—Aichmophobia; Xyrophobia
Red—Erythrophobia
Relationships, close—Philophobia
Remembering—Mnemophobia
Responsibility, assuming—Hypengyophobia
Ridicule-Catagelophobia
Right side of body, objects on—Dextrophobia
Rituals, religious—Hagiophobia
Rivers—Potamophobia
Robbed, being—Clepto-; Kleptophobia
Robbers—Harpaxophobia
Rope—Linonophobia
Ruins—Ate-; Atophobia
Sacred things, places—Hagiophobia; Hierophobia
Saltiness—Halophobia
Scabies—Scabiophobia
School—Epistemophobia
Scratched, being—Amychophobia
Sea—Thalassophobia; Pelagophobia
Seated, being—Thaasophobia
Self-destructive actions—Ergasiophobia
Semen—Spermatophobia
Sexual excitement—Ceratophobia
Sexual identity—Genophobia
Sexual intercourse—Coitophobia; Erotophobia
Sexual organs: Of either sex—Genitophobia;
         Female—Eurotiphobia
Sharks—Selachophobia
Sharp objects—Aichmophobia
Sharp (sour) tastes—Acerbo-; Acerophobia
Shock—Hormephobia (see Electrophobia, fear of electricity)
Sin—Hamartophobia

Sinning—Peccatiphobia
Sitting down—Kathisophobia
Skin—Dermatophobia
Skin diseases—Dermatopathophobia; Dermatosiophobia
Sleep—Hypnophobia
Small insects—Acarophobia
Stinging insects—Melissophobia
Small objects—Microphobia
Smothered, being—Pnigero-; Pnigophobia
Snakes—Ophidiophobia
Snow—Chionophobia
Society, human—Anthro-; Anthropophobia
Solitude—Autophobia; Eremiophobia; Monophobia
Sounds, various—Acousticophobia; Phonophobia
Sour tastes—Acerbo-; Acerophobia
Space, outer—Astrophobia; Stratophobia
Spaces:
       Confined—Claustrophobia
       Empty—Kenophobia; Topophobia
       Open—Agoraphobia
Speaking (in public)—Lalio-; Lalophobia
Spiders—Arachneo-; Arachnophobia
Spirits, evil—Daemono-; Demonophobia; Phasmophobia
Staircases—Climacophobia
Standing and walking—Stabisbasiphobia
Standing upright—Stasiphobia
Stared at, being—Ophthalmophobia; Scopophobia
Stars—Siderophobia
Statues—Pediophobia
Stealing—Clepto-; Kleptophobia
Sticks—Rhabdophobia
Strangeness—Neophobia
Strangers—Xenophobia
Streets, crossing—Agyiophobia
String—Linonophobia
Stuttering—Lalio-; Lalophobia

Success—Chrysophobia
Suicide—Ergasiophobia
Sunshine—Heliophobia
Sweetness (taste)—Hediso-; Hedysophobia
Syphilis—Syphilophobia; Cypridophobia; Venereophobia
Tapeworms—Taeniophobia
Tastes, various—Geumatophobia
        (see also list under "Flavors")
Teeth—Odontophobia
Tetanus—Tetanophobia
Theft, thieves—Clepto-; Kleptophobia; Harpaxophobia
Thinking—Phronemophobia
Thirteen (number)—Triskaidekaphobia
Time, passage of—Chronophobia
Thunder—Brontophobia; Tonitrophobia
        (see Astraphobia; Keraunophobia, fear of lightning)
Tornadoes—Anemophobia
Touched, being—Aphe-; Haphe-; Haptephobia
Trains, travel by—Siderodromophobia
Travel—Hodophobia
Trees—Dendrophobia
Trembling—Tremophobia
Trichinosis—Trichinophobia
Tuberculosis—Phthisiophobia; Tuberculophobia
Twins—Didymophobia
Ugliness—Cacho-; Cacophobia
Uncleanliness, personal—Automysophobia
Untidiness—Ataxiophobia; Auchmophobia; Conistraphobia
Vaccination—Vaccino; Vaccophobia
Vapors-Aerophobia
Vehicle, being in—Amaxophobia
Venereal diseases—Cyprido-; Cypriphobia; Syphilophobia;
        Venereophobia
Vomiting—Emetophobia
Voids—Kenophobia; Topophobia
Walking—Basi-; Basophobia

Wandering about—Dromophobia
War—Polemophobia
Watched, being—Ophthalmophobia; Scopophobia
Watches—Chronophobia
Water:

        General—Hydrophobia
        Deep-Batho-; Bathyphobia
        Flowing—Potamophobia
        Large bodies of—Potaniophobia

Weakness, physical—Asthenophobia
Wealth—Chrysophobia
White—Leucophobia
Winds, high—Anemophobia
Wind instruments—Aulophobia
Wolves—Lycophobia
Women—Gynephobia
Work—Ergophobia; Ponophobia
Worms—Helminthophobia
Writing (in public)—Graphophobia
Yellow—Xanthophobia

APPENDIX C

What To Do If A Family Member Has An Anxiety Disorder [1]

1) Don't make assumptions about what the affected person needs. Ask them.

2) Be predictable. Don't surprise them.

3) Let the person with the disorder set the pace for recovery.

4) Find something positive in every experience. If the affected person is only able to go part way to a particular goal, such as a movie theater or party, consider that an achievement rather than a failure.

5) Don't enable avoidance. Negotiate with the person with panic disorder to take one step forward when he or she wants to avoid something.

6) Don't sacrifice your own life and build resentments.

7) Don't panic when the person with the disorder panics.

8) Remember that it's all right to be anxious yourself. It's natural for you to be concerned and even worried about the person with panic disorder.

9) Be patient and accepting but don't settle for the affected person being permanently disabled.

10) Say: "You can do it no matter how you feel. I am proud of you. Tell me what you need now. Breathe slow and low. Stay in the present. It's not the place that's bothering you, it's the thought. I know that what you are feeling is painful, but it's not dangerous. You are courageous.

11) Don't say: "Relax. Calm down. Don't be anxious. Let's see if you can do this (i.e., setting up a test for the affected person). You can fight this. What should we do next? Don't be ridiculous. You HAVE to stay. Don't be a coward."

APPENDIX - D

More information is available by writing to or calling:

1. American Psychiatric Association
    1400 K Street, NW
    Washington, D.C. 20005
    (202) 682-6000
    (202) 682-6850 Fax
    www.psych.org/
    E-Mail - apa@psych.org

2. American Psychological Association
    750 First Street, N.E.
    Washington, D.C. 20002-4242
    (202) 336-5500
    www.apa.org
    E-Mail - go to www.apa.org/about/contact.html

3. Anxiety Disorders of America 1999
    11900 Parklawn Drive, Suite 100
    Rockville, MD 20852
    (301) 231-9350
    www.adaa.org/
    E-Mail - anxdis@adaa.org

4. Association for the Advancement of Behavior Therapy
    305 Seventh Avenue - 16th Floor
    New York, NY 10001-6008
    (212) 647-1890
    (212) 647-1865 Fax
    http://server.psyc.vt.edu/aabt/

5. National Alliance for the Mentally Ill
    200 North Glebe Road, Suite 1015
    Arlington, VA 22203-3754
    Helpline: 1-800-950-6264
    Front Desk: (703) 524-7600
    TDD - (703)516-7227
    Fax - (703) 524-9094
    www.nami.org/
    E-Mail - helpline@nami.org

6. National Anxiety Foundation
    3135 Custer Drive
    Lexington, KY 40517-4001
    www.lexington-on-line.com/naf.html

7. National Depressive/Manic Depressive Assn.
    730 North Franklin Street, Suite 501
    Chicago, IL 60610-3526
    1-800-826-3632
    (312)642-7243 Fax
    www.ndmda.org/
    E-Mail - myrtis@aol.com

8. National Institute of Mental Health
    NIMH Public Inquiries
    6001 Executive Blvd.
    Room 8184 MSC 9663
    Bethesda MD 20892-9663
    www.nimh.nih.gov/
    E-Mail - nimhinfo@nih.gov

9. Mental Health Information Center
    1-800-969-6642
    (703) 684-5968 Fax
    TTY Line 800-433-5959
    www.nmha.org/

10.   National Mental Health Association
      1021 Prince Street
      Alexandria, VA 22314-2971
      (703) 684-7722

11.   Free brochures on Panic Disorders and its treatment,
      Call: 1-888-8-ANXIETY

12.   Panic Disorder Education Program
      5600 Fishers Ln., Rm. 7C-02, msc 8030
      Bethesda, MD 20892
      Office: (301) 443-4536
      FAX: (301) 443-0008

13.   Ross Center for Anxiety and Related Disorders
      4545 42nd St., NW, Suite 311
      Washington, D.C. 20016
      (202) 363-1010
      www.rosscenter.com/index.cfm
      To contact go to
      www.rosscenter.com/contact.cfm

FOOTNOTES

Chapter Two

1. Robert Handly with Pauline Neff, Anxiety & Panic Attacks—
   Their Cause and Cure (New York: Rawson Associates, 1985),
   pp.21-22.

Chapter Three

1. Arthur B. Hardy, M.D., "Rationale for the Origin of
   Agoraphobia," booklet entitled Agoraphobia Symptoms,
   Causes, Treatment (1976).

2. Ibid.

3. National Institute of Mental Health: Panic Disorder,
   DHHS Publ. No. (ADM) 91-1869 (Washington, D.C.: U.S. Dept.
   of Health & Human Services, 1991).

4. American Psychiatric Association: Diagnostic and Statistical
   Manual of Mental Disorders, Third Ed., Revised (Washington,
   D.C.: American Psychiatric Association, 1987), p.238.

5. Natl. Institute...: Panic Disorder, op.cit.

6. Am. Psychiatric...: Diagnostic and..., op.cit., p. 238.

7. Natl. Institute...: Panic Disorder, op.cit.

Chapter Six

1. Leo Buscaglia, Ph.D., Living, Loving & Learning, Steven Short, ed. (USA: Charles B. Slack, 1982), pp. 5-6.

2. Leo Buscaglia, Love (New York: Ballantine Books, 1972), pp. 9-11.

3. Buscaglia, Living..., op.cit., pp. 263-264.

Chapter Seven

1. Fraser Kent, Nothing to Fear—Coping with Phobias (New York: Doubleday Company, 1977), Appendix, pp. 180-190.

Chapter Ten

1. Tudi Pleban, "Positive Affirmations," especially written for her sister, Patty, for Flight 201, U.S. Air, Pittsburgh to Orlando (1993).

2. Don and Nancy Tubesing, Relax—Let Go—Relax, Mary O'Brien Sippel, RN, MS and Donald A. Tubesing, Ph.D., narrators (USA: Whole Person Associates).

3. Prayer to St. Joseph, The Pieta Prayer Booklet (USA: Miraculous Lady of the Roses, 1992), p. 17.

4. Larry Henley and Jeff Silbar, Wind Beneath My Wings (Published by W B Gold Music Corp., ASCAP/Warner House of Music, BMI, 1982).

Appendix - B

Phobias Listed by Objects of Fear

1. Fraser Kent, Nothing to Fear—Coping with Phobias (New York: Doubleday & Company, 1977), Appendix, pp. 180-190.

Appendix - C

1. Adapted from Sally Winston, Psy.D., The Anxiety and Stress Disorders Institute of Maryland, Towson, Md., 1992.
   National Institute of Mental Health booklet, NIMH Panic Disorder Education Program, "Understanding Panic Disorder."
   NIH No. 93-3509 (1993), p.11.